AF880785

A PHOTOGRAPHIC JOURNEY THROUGH THE WORK OF ANESTHESIOLOGIST

THE LIFE SAVERS

THE INVISIBLE WORLD OF ANESTHESIOLOGY

Author

Prof. Admir Hadzic, MD, PhD

NYSORA® PRESS

Publishing Division of NYSORA, Inc
2585 Broadway, suite 183, New York, NY10025
info@nysora.com, www.nysora.com

Copyright 2026 by Nysora, Inc. All rights reserved. No part of this publication can be reproduced or distributed in any form or by any means, or stored in a database or retrieval system, without the prior written permission of the publisher.

Library of Congress Identification
Authors: Prof. Admir Hadzic, MD, PhD
Title: THE LIFE SAVERS
Subtitle: The Invisible World of Anesthesiology
2026 Edition
Identifiers:
Library of Congress Control Number: 2026901191
ISBN: 978-1-966637-14-1

Table of Contents

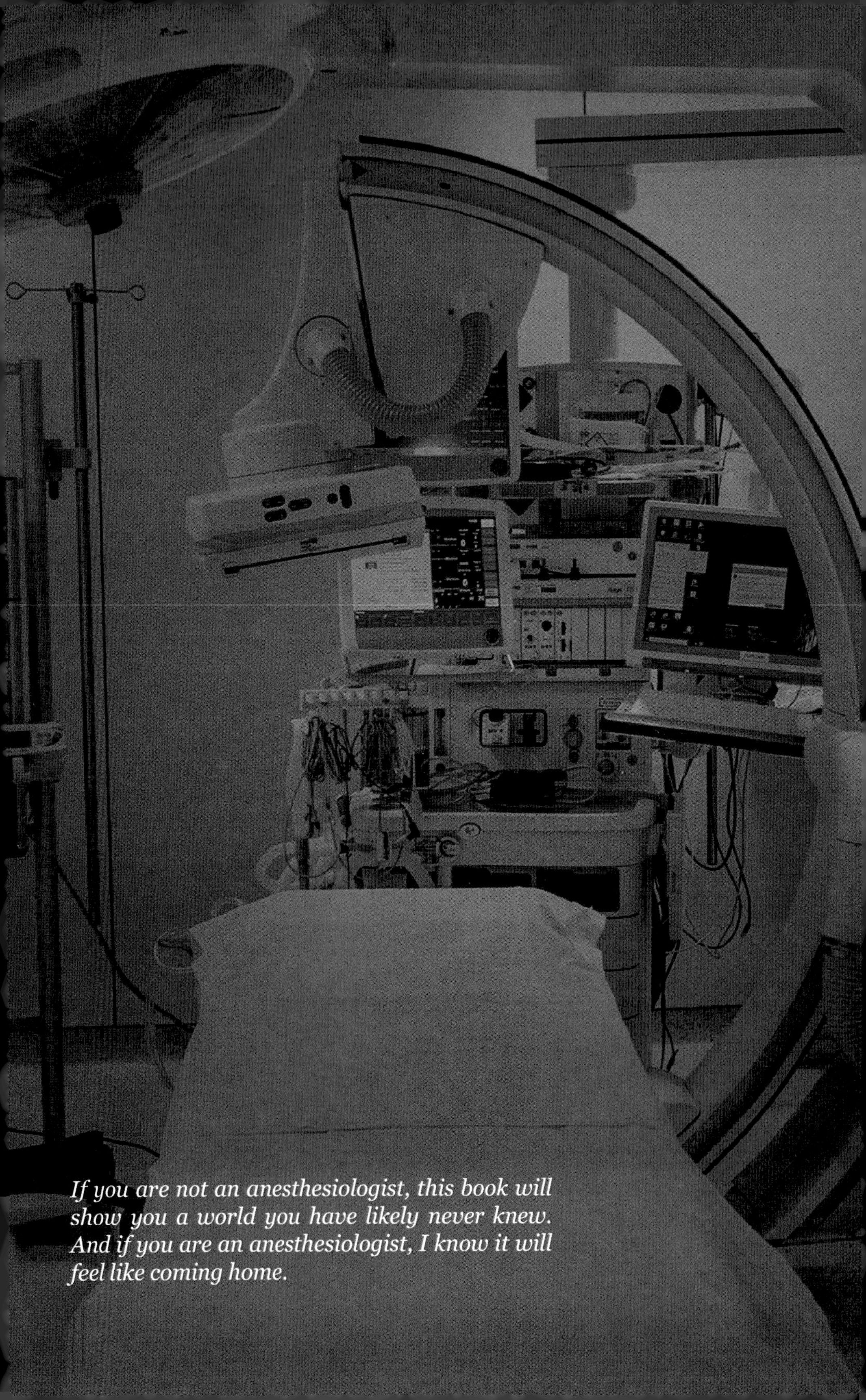

If you are not an anesthesiologist, this book will show you a world you have likely never knew. And if you are an anesthesiologist, I know it will feel like coming home.

Prologue

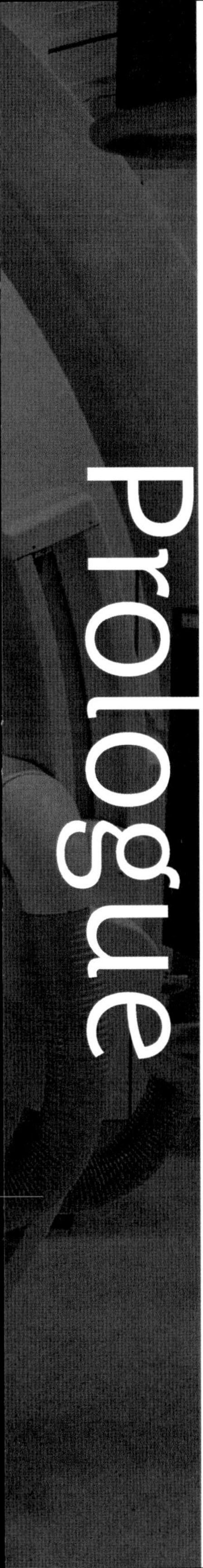

The Empty Operating Room

The operating room is always deceivingly quiet in the morning. Before anyone arrives, it looks almost peaceful; an empty OR table, neatly draped instruments, a ventilator standing still, screens dark or idling. The operating room schedule was printed yesterday. The cases look routine. On paper, the day appears controllable. But everyone who has ever practiced anesthesia knows the truth: Nothing about this room is routine. Even after decades, I still pause for a second at the door any time I pass by an operating room, because the look through the OR window is rarely reflective on what was written on the schedule a day before. Never a routine.

Anesthesia begins long before the first incision. It starts in silence: checking the oxygen supply, testing the suction, running a hand over the breathing circuit, and making sure the equipment is fully operational, medication drawers, reading the patient's history as if it were a weather forecast. The room is always cold in a way only operating rooms manage to be, and the first scent that tells you you're not here for the morning coffee, it's disinfectant: chlorhexidine, plastic, and something metallic you stop noticing only when you're no longer paying attention.

You learn to recognize patterns the way sailors read the sea. A small detail, a note in patient's record about sleep apnea, a vague comment about "difficult intubation," a medication that suggests heart failure, can change everything. To an outside observer, it might look like preparation for something simple: put the patient to sleep, keep them asleep during the operation, wake them up when it's done.

In reality, however, anesthesiology is the art and science of guiding a living human through a controlled physiologic storm. The moment the patient enters, the room changes. The quiet fills with voices, equipment noise, the hasty rhythm of opening surgical equipment, anesthesia medications and preparation for airway management.

The rhythm of beeping monitors begins like a metronome desynced into an unpredictable polyphony. A cacophony of noises of the OR staff coordinating. Cables multiply. Tubing creeps in from everywhere. A suction canister sits on the floor, and the wet, rhythmic pull from the surgical field fills the room. Infusion pumps wake up. A blood pressure cuff cycles. The pulse oximeter finds its signal. Numbers populate the screen, heart rate, reads oxygen saturation, end-tidal CO_2, tidal volumes, pressures, temperatures. Each one a tiny information snippet, combined in a language you spend years learning to read and understand. And then the drapes go up and the operation starts. From that moment on, the patient becomes invisible to most of the room. The surgeon sees a field. The assistants see instruments. The nurse sees workflow.

But the anesthesiologist sees the person who can no longer speak for themselves: whose breathing, blood pressure, body temperature and bare survival have been handed over in trust.

That trust is quiet. It isn't the kind that comes with applause. It's not even the kind that gets noticed when it is working. It is simply assumed. The best way I could describe it.

Anesthetizing a patient is often described as flying a plane: takeoff and landing are what matter; everything in between is routine. I have always found that comparison logical for everyone except us, the anesthesiologists. Because in anesthesia, there is no autopilot.

Every small manual, experienced-based adjustment matters. A faster IV fluid flow. A few micrograms of an IV medication or infusion. A slight change in ventilation. Concentration of inhalational anesthetic gas. Level of muscle paralysis and relaxation. Airway pressures and end-tidal CO_2 information. Constantly making decisions to which the patient responds immediately, sometimes predictably, sometimes with a physiology you do not expect. Sometimes a response you've never seen before. Two people can undergo the same anesthetic and surgical intervention and respond like entirely different species. That is

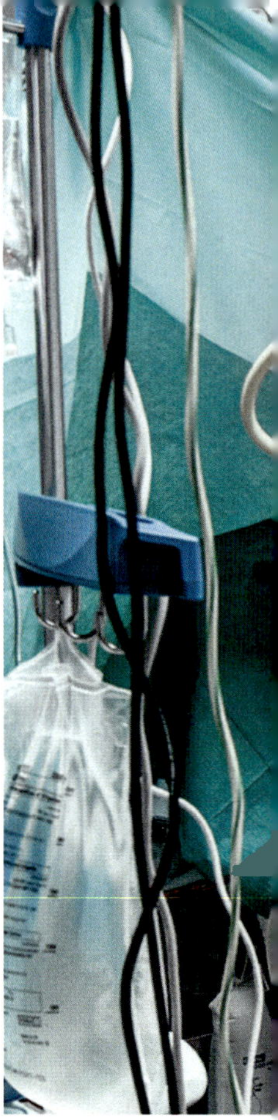

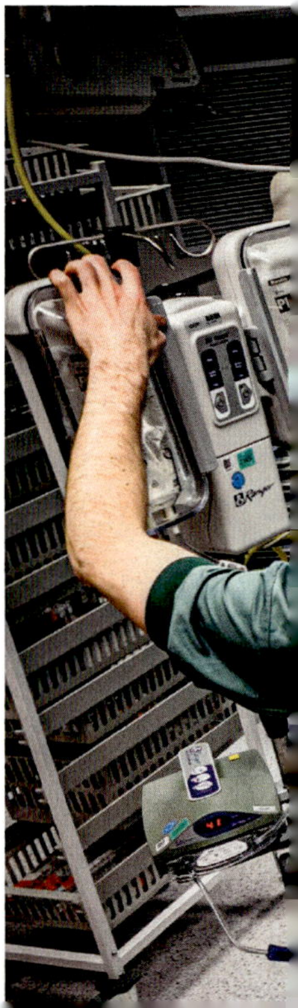

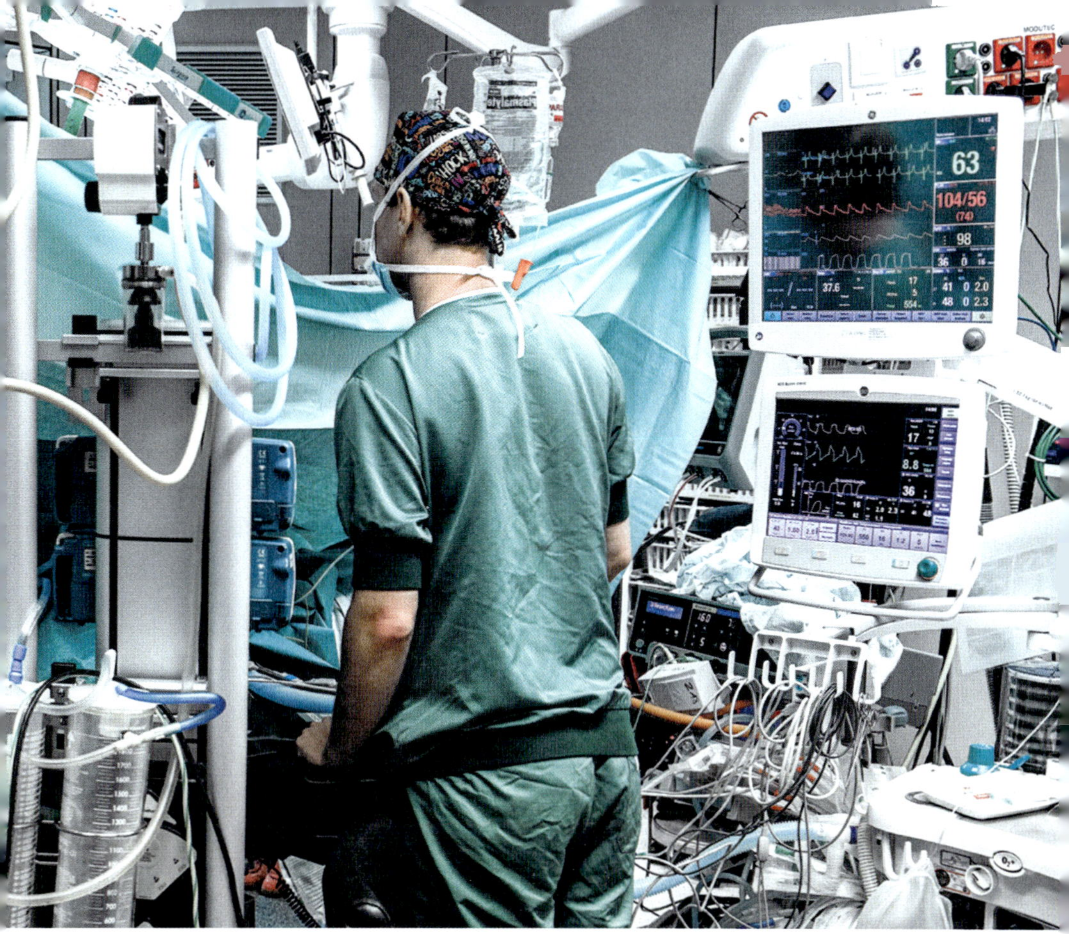
63
104/56
(74)
98

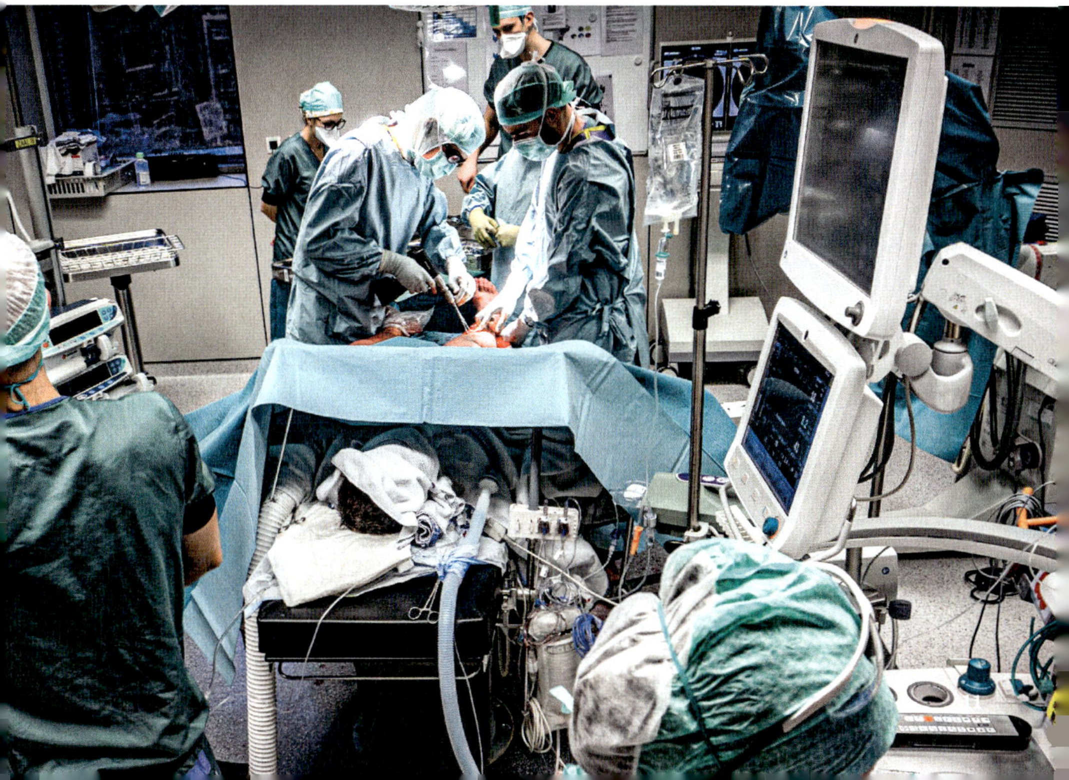

what makes practicing anesthesiology challenging, and what makes it deeply human. It is also what makes it lonely at times. Paradoxically, you are always surrounded by a team, yet much of your work happens only in your head: anticipating bleeding before it arrives, treating hypotension before it becomes dangerous, seeing a trend before it becomes a crisis. You learn to stay calm when everyone else can't, and to keep calm and focused while doing several things at once.

Sometimes the only sound at your end of the OR table is the rhythm of the breathing machine cycling-steady, indifferent, predictable. There's been times when after years of practicing anesthesiology I asked myself standing at the head of the table, surrounded by life-sustaining equipment: "Is this real"? Am I really here, and would this person really die if I slipped up? The immense jolt of responsibility reminds you how physical the "invisible" work of being anesthesiologist really is.

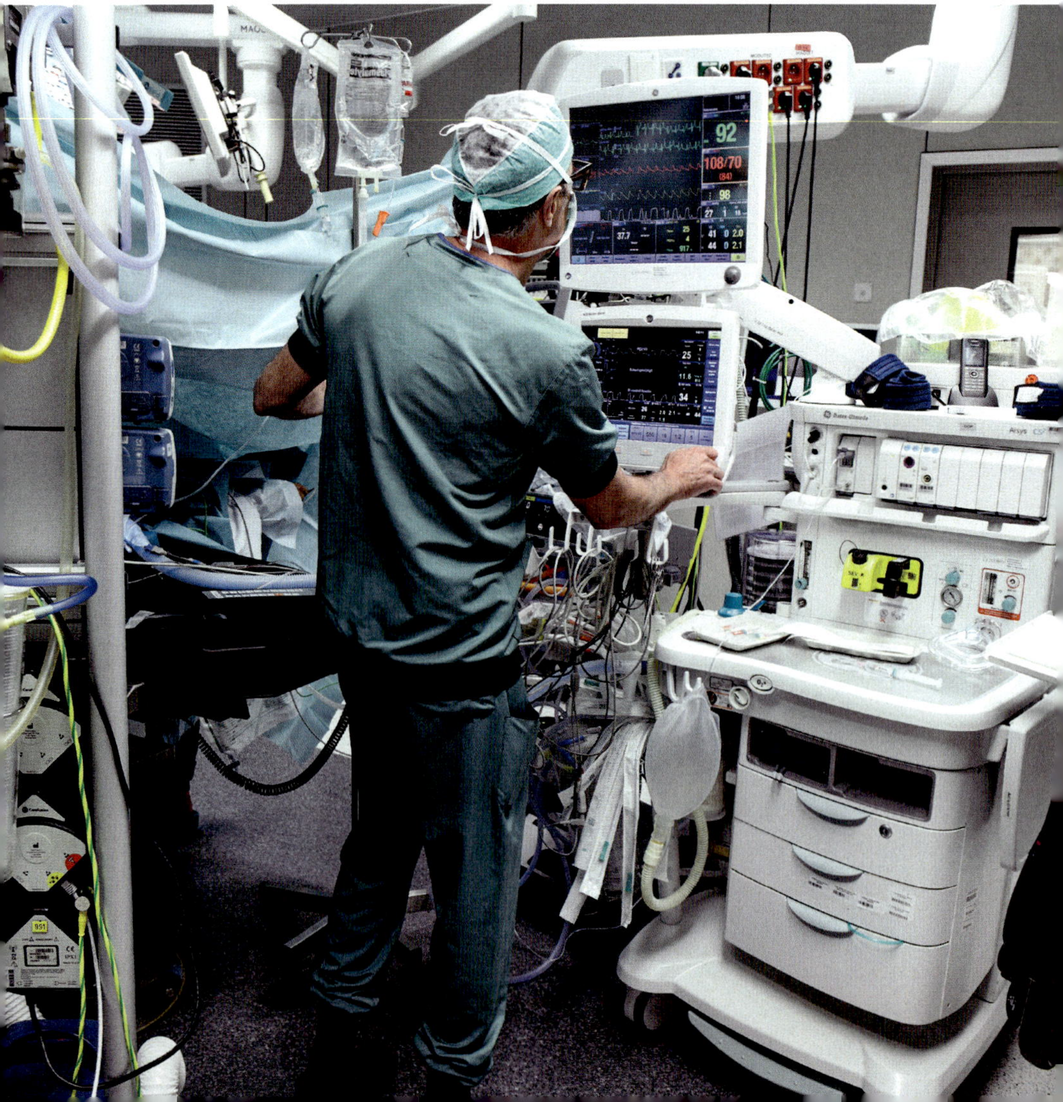

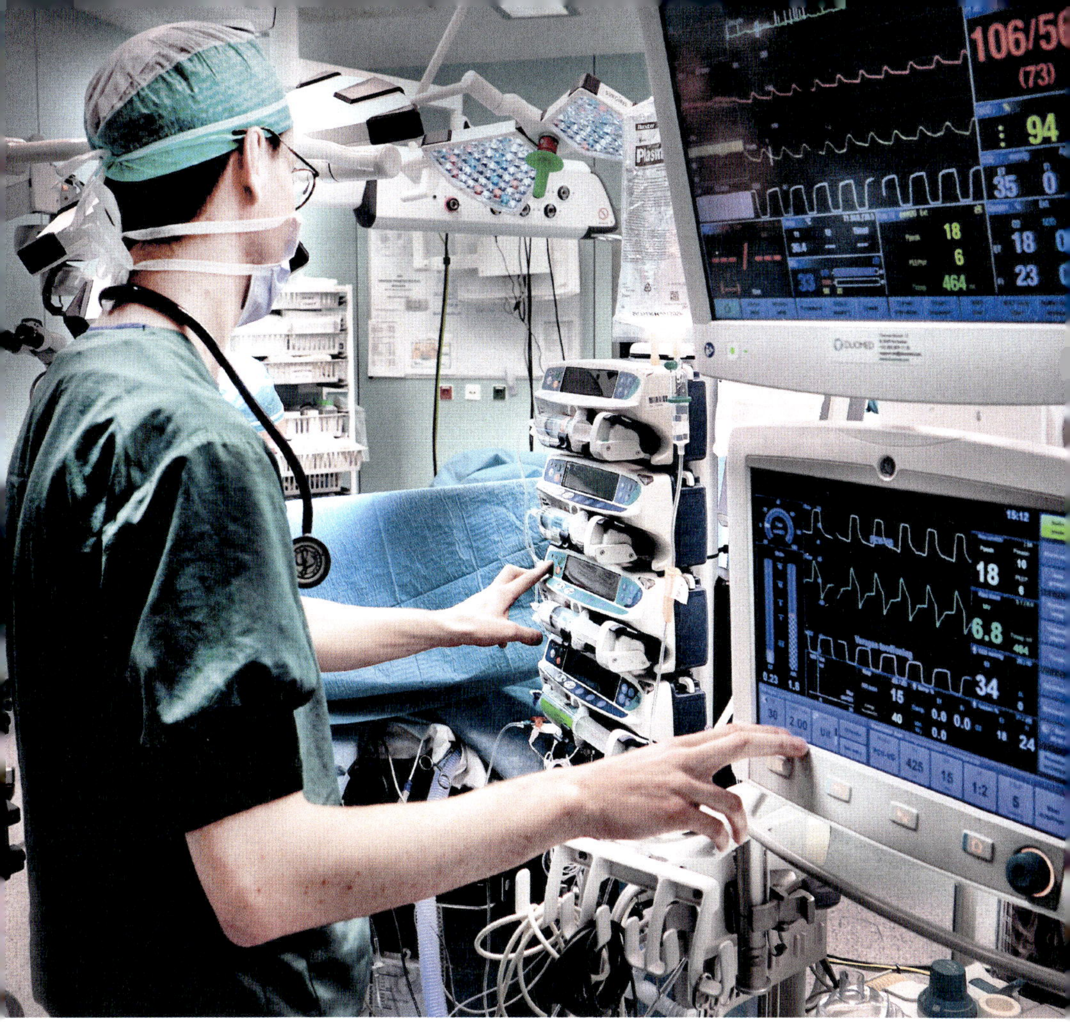

When it goes well, it looks like nothing happened. And that is the point.

Over more than three decades, I have lived thousands of days like this: early mornings, late nights, holiday shifts, cases that ended routinely, and cases that changed a life forever. Along the way, I took notes and photographed what I saw: not the theatrical moments that press loves to display, but the real ones: hands steady at the airway, eyes fixed on a waveform, a quiet pause before induction. The choreography of a team taking care of a highly vulnerable human being without speaking.

I started documenting these moments because I realized how much of our work disappears the instant it succeeds. This book is not a textbook, nor is it a catalogue of heroics. It is a photographic journey through the unseen life of anesthesiologists: the stillness before the storm, the vigilance during it, the responsibility carried without spectacle, the humor we use to survive it, and the strange privilege of being the person whose job is to keep a heartbeat going often against all odds.

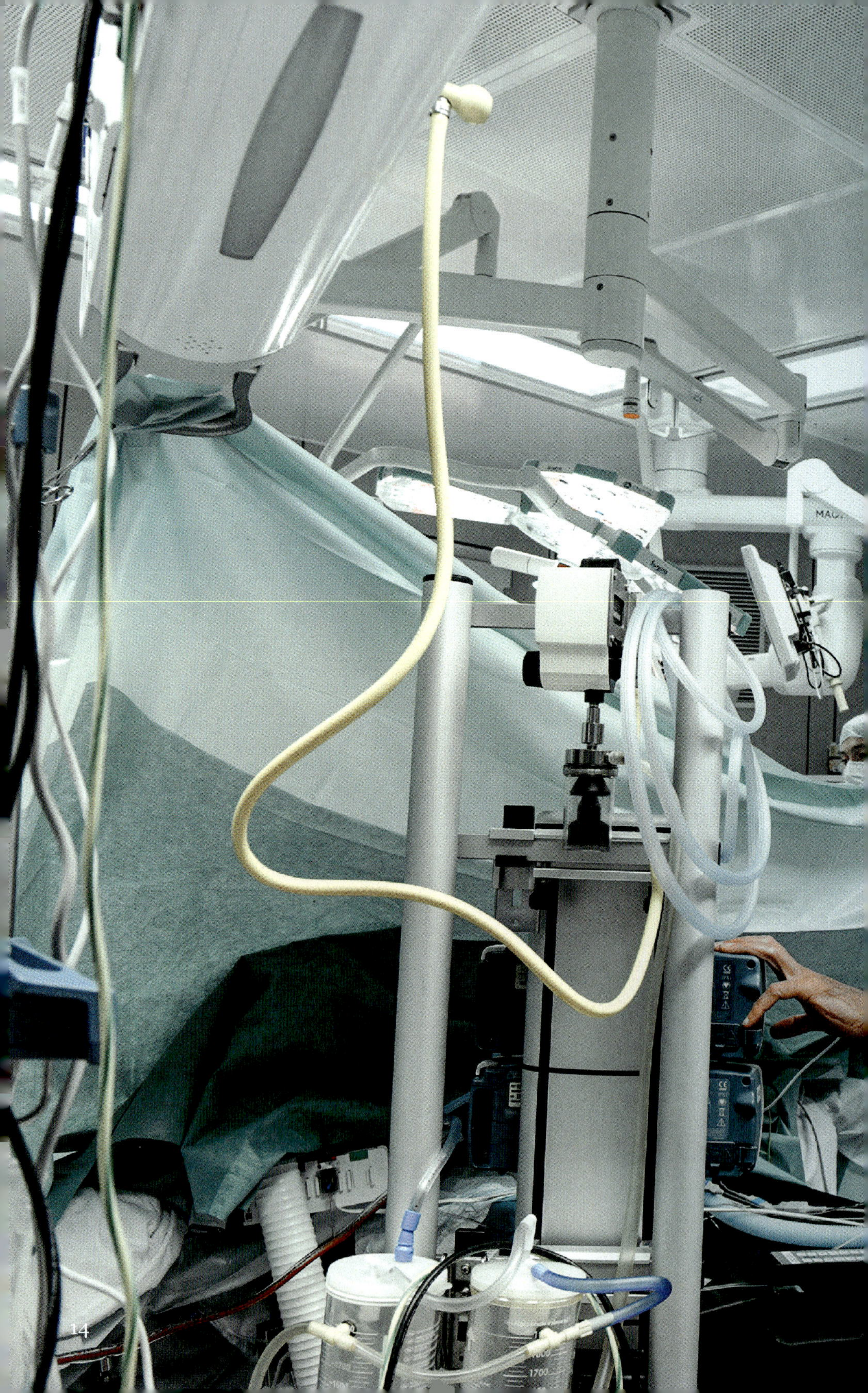

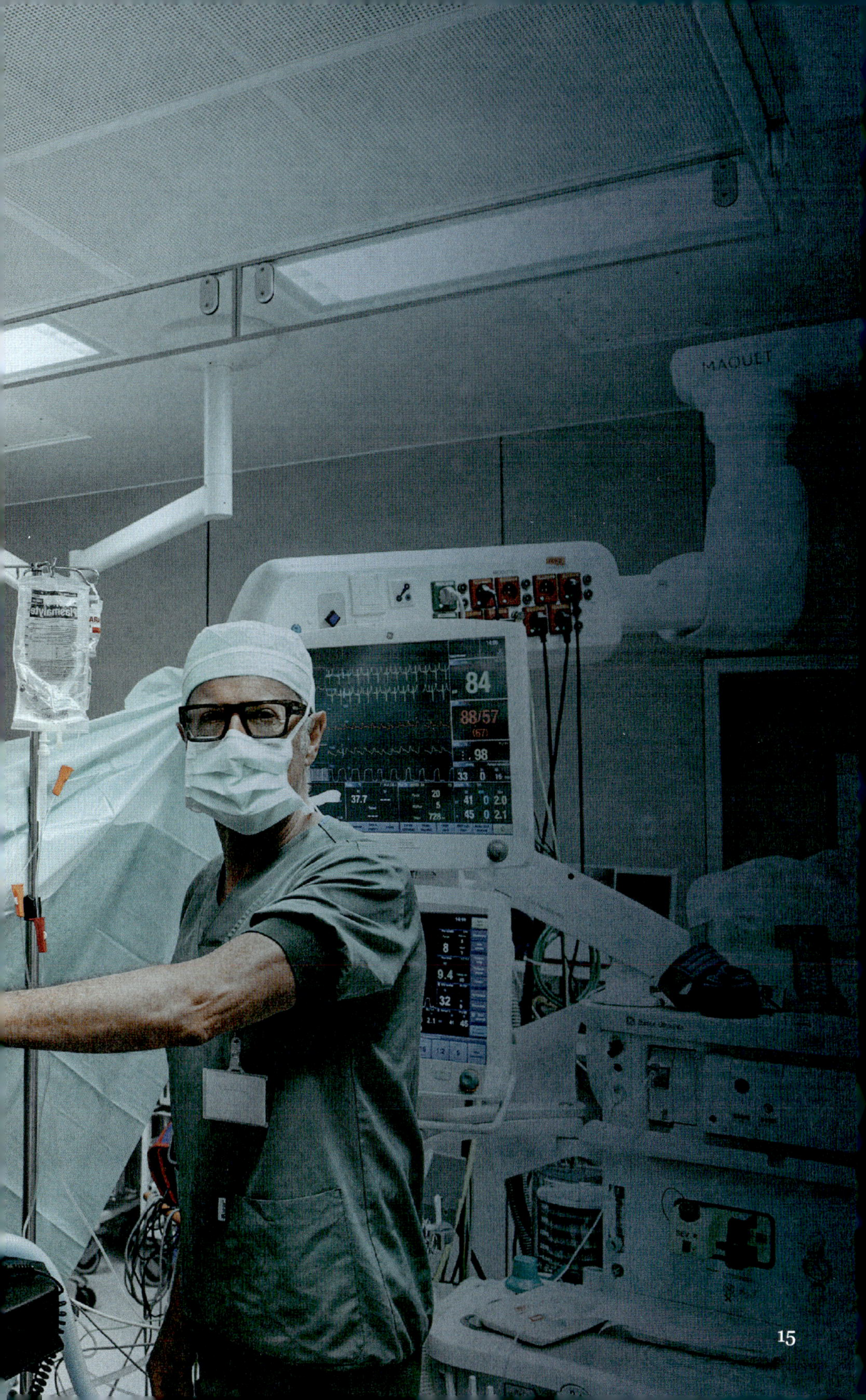
MAQUET
84
88/57
(67)
98

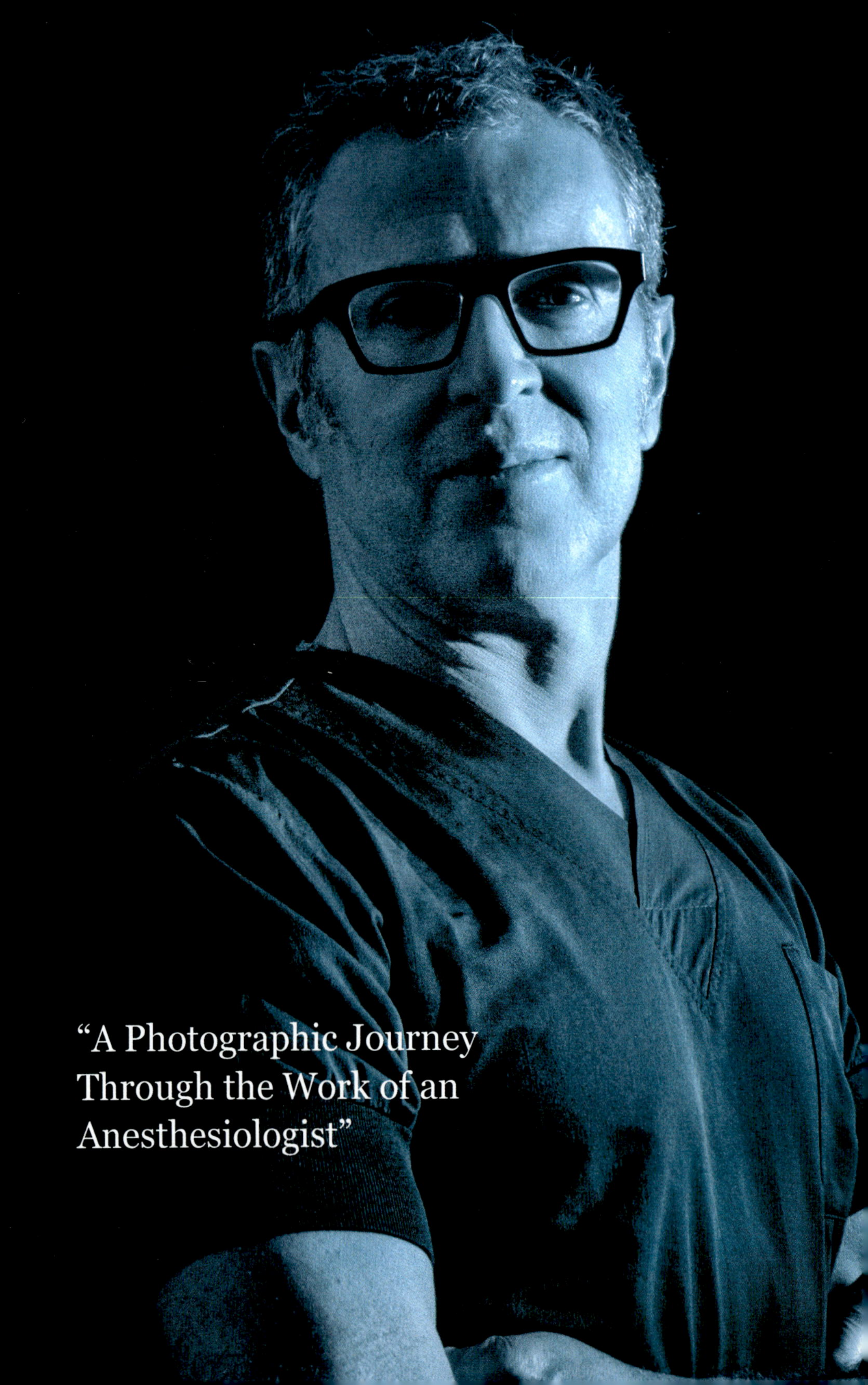
"A Photographic Journey Through the Work of an Anesthesiologist"

Introduction

What This Book Is - and What It Is Not

Most people meet anesthesiologists at a vulnerable moment. They meet us briefly, often minutes before surgery, when anxiety is high and time feels compressed. We introduce ourselves, ask a few questions, explain just enough to establish trust and then we take that trust with us behind the drapes. When everything goes well, we disappear again. When it doesn't, we are suddenly impossible to ignore.

For many patients, that is the entire relationship. This book exists because that narrow window does not reflect the reality of anesthesiology. Anesthesiologists do not simply "put people to sleep." We manage physiology in its most fragile states. We work at the intersection of medicine, surgery, technology, and human judgment. We make decisions continuously, often invisibly, and we do so in moments where errors are unforgiving and success leaves no trace.

And yet, despite its central role in modern medicine, anesthesiology remains poorly understood: by the public, by students, and sometimes even by our medical colleagues. This book is an attempt to change that. It is not a textbook. It is not a history of anesthesia.

And it is not a collection of heroic OR war stories.

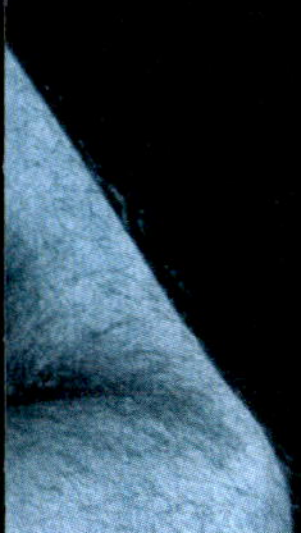

Instead, it is an honest visual and narrative exploration of what anesthesiology actually is: a profession defined by focus, restraint, preparation, and responsibility. A craft practiced in silence. A specialty where excellence often looks like nothing happening at all. I have practiced anesthesiology for almost three decades. Over that time, I took photographs and notes about anesthesiologists in action. Quiet moments. Tense moments. Eyes fixed on a waveform, hands steady at an airway, a pause before induction. The actions of anesthesiologists and nurses, a team that knows each other well enough not to speak.

What emerged was an amazing realization that much of our work vanishes the instant it succeeds. This book is a response to that disappearance. The chapters that follow move through the life of anesthesiology, from the empty operating room at dawn, to the loneliness of holiday shifts, to the discipline required when treating VIP patients, to the moment when anesthesiologists themselves become patients. Along the way, it explores the questions people rarely ask out loud: Is anesthesia dangerous? Why one becomes an anesthesiologist? What kind of person thrives in this role? Some chapters are reflective. Others are instructional. But all are grounded in lived experience.

If you are not an anesthesiologist, this book will show you a world that has likely protected you without ever introducing itself. You may never look at surgery and anesthesia quite the same way again.

If you are a medical student or trainee, this book is meant to inform you honestly: Anesthesiology is not for everyone. Understanding that early is essential.

And if you are an anesthesiologist, you will recognize yourself here. The responsibility you carry: quietly, every day, finally seen by outside world.

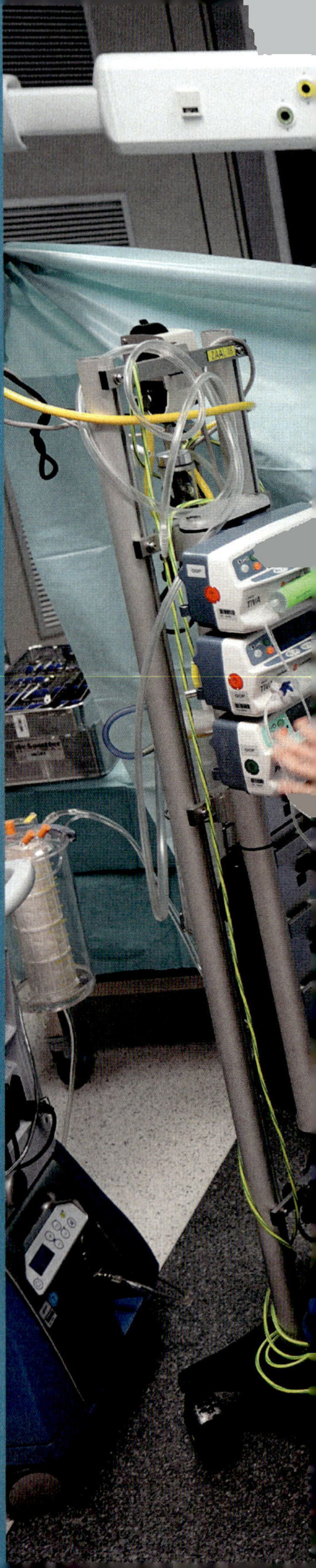

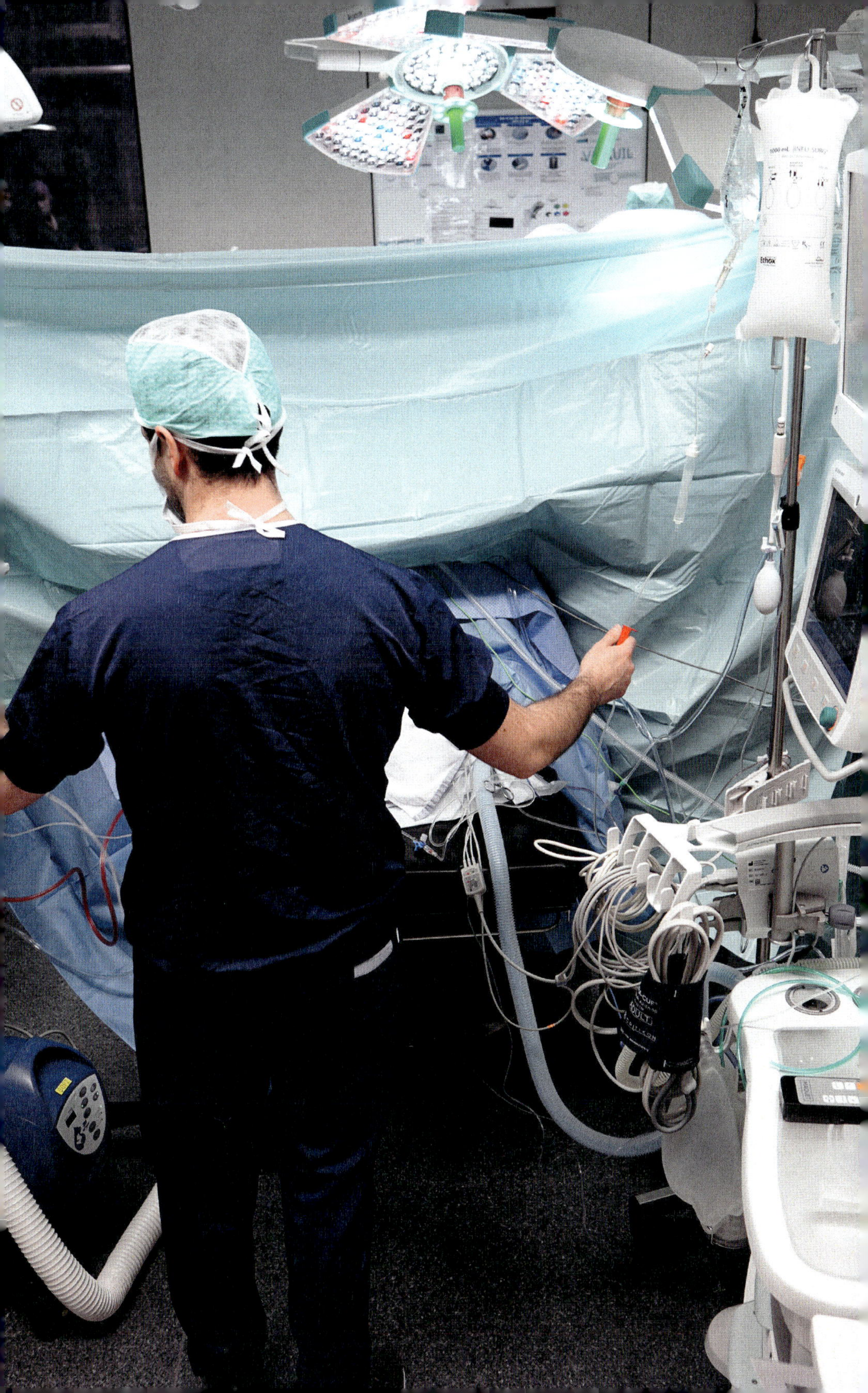
Ethox

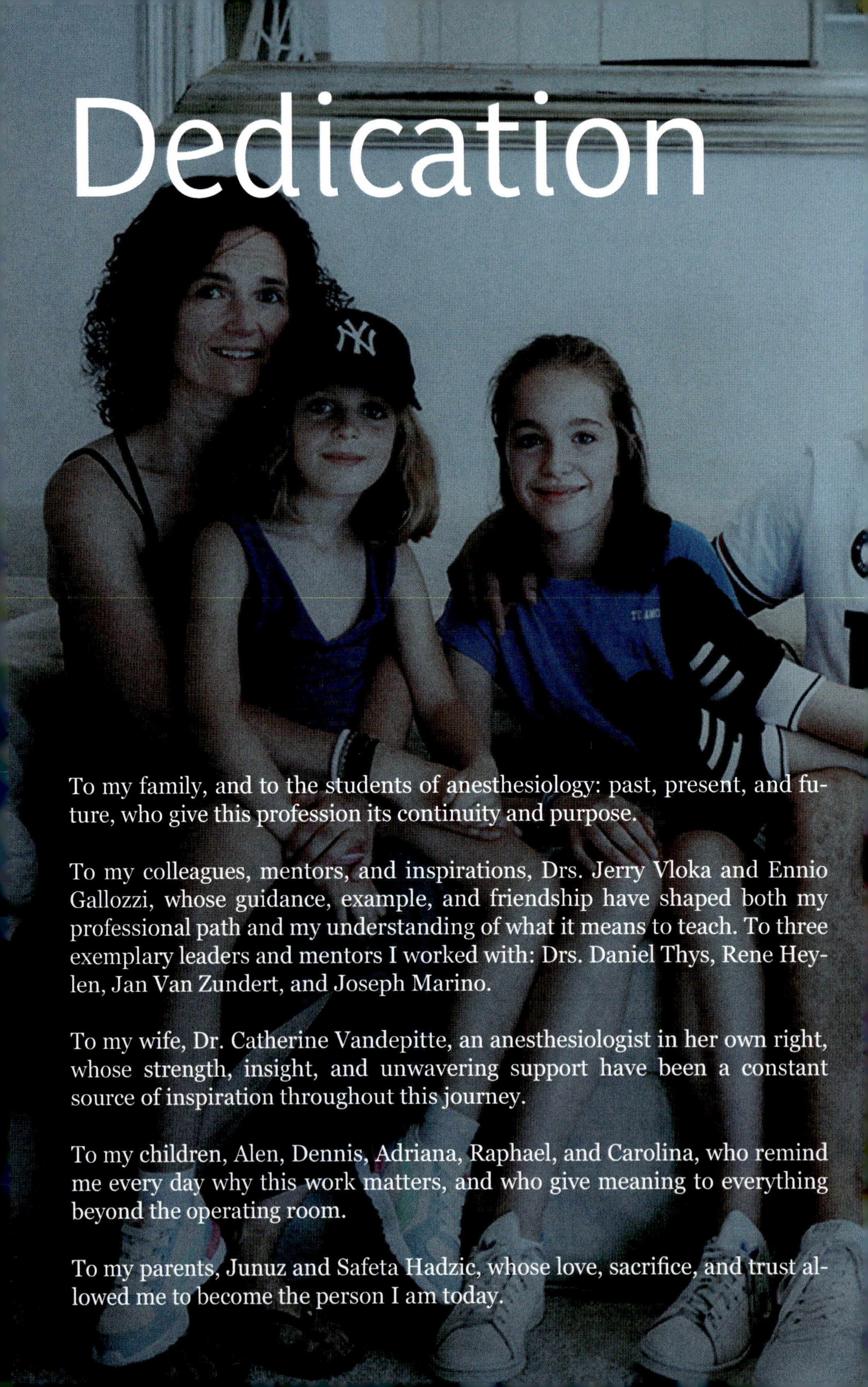

Dedication

To my family, and to the students of anesthesiology: past, present, and future, who give this profession its continuity and purpose.

To my colleagues, mentors, and inspirations, Drs. Jerry Vloka and Ennio Gallozzi, whose guidance, example, and friendship have shaped both my professional path and my understanding of what it means to teach. To three exemplary leaders and mentors I worked with: Drs. Daniel Thys, Rene Heylen, Jan Van Zundert, and Joseph Marino.

To my wife, Dr. Catherine Vandepitte, an anesthesiologist in her own right, whose strength, insight, and unwavering support have been a constant source of inspiration throughout this journey.

To my children, Alen, Dennis, Adriana, Raphael, and Carolina, who remind me every day why this work matters, and who give meaning to everything beyond the operating room.

To my parents, Junuz and Safeta Hadzic, whose love, sacrifice, and trust allowed me to become the person I am today.

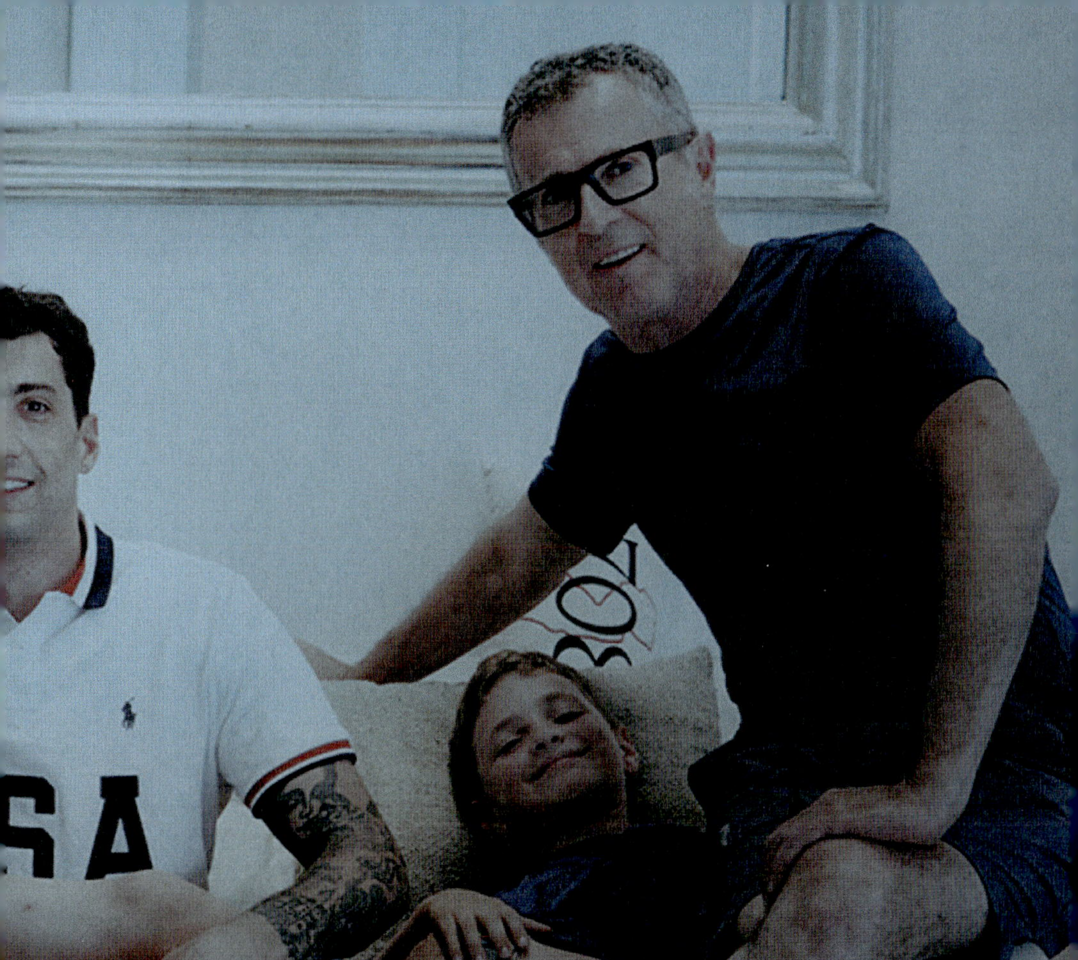

To my colleagues and friends at St. Luke's - Roosevelt Hospital in New York, ZOL Genk in Belgium, and Northwell University Hospital at North Shore, New York, with whom I have shared responsibility, learning, and the quiet moments that define our profession.

To my NYSORA team of dedicated educators, designers, filmmakers, and innovators, whose creativity, discipline, and belief in education make everything NYSORA does possible.

And finally, to my academic homes: Karol Marcinkowski, Poznan University of Medical Sciences where I earned my PhD under the mentorship of Professor Leon Drobnik and where I am honored to hold an honorary title of Doctor Honoris Causa Dr. h.c. (Honorary title of Doctor Honoris Causa) the University of Ljubljana, Slovenia, where I hold an honorary professorship; and the Catholic University of Leuven, whose Department of Anesthesiology I am privileged to serve as a Visiting professor.

This book belongs to all of you.

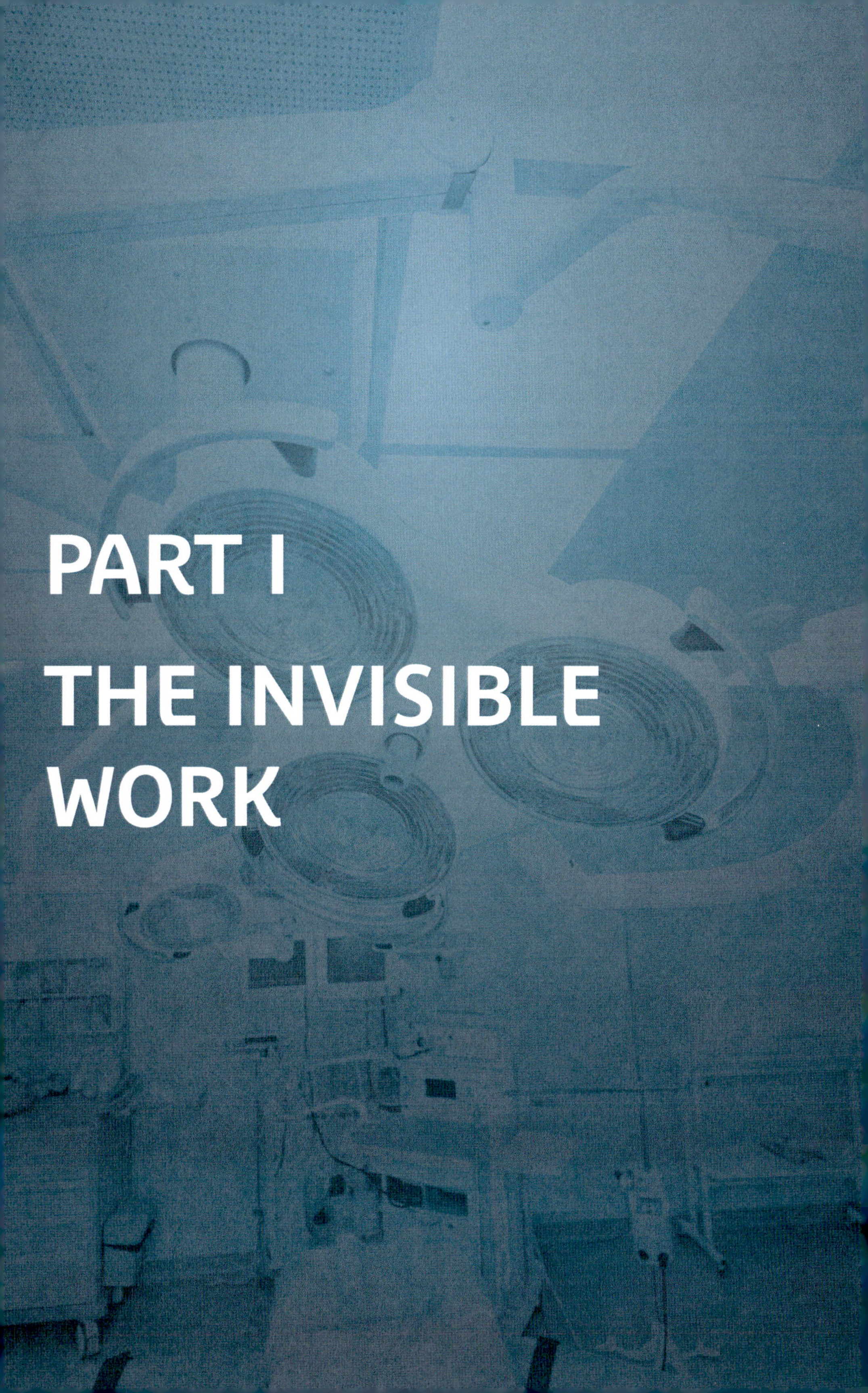

PART I

THE INVISIBLE WORK

Chapter 1

Behind the Drapes - The Work No One Sees

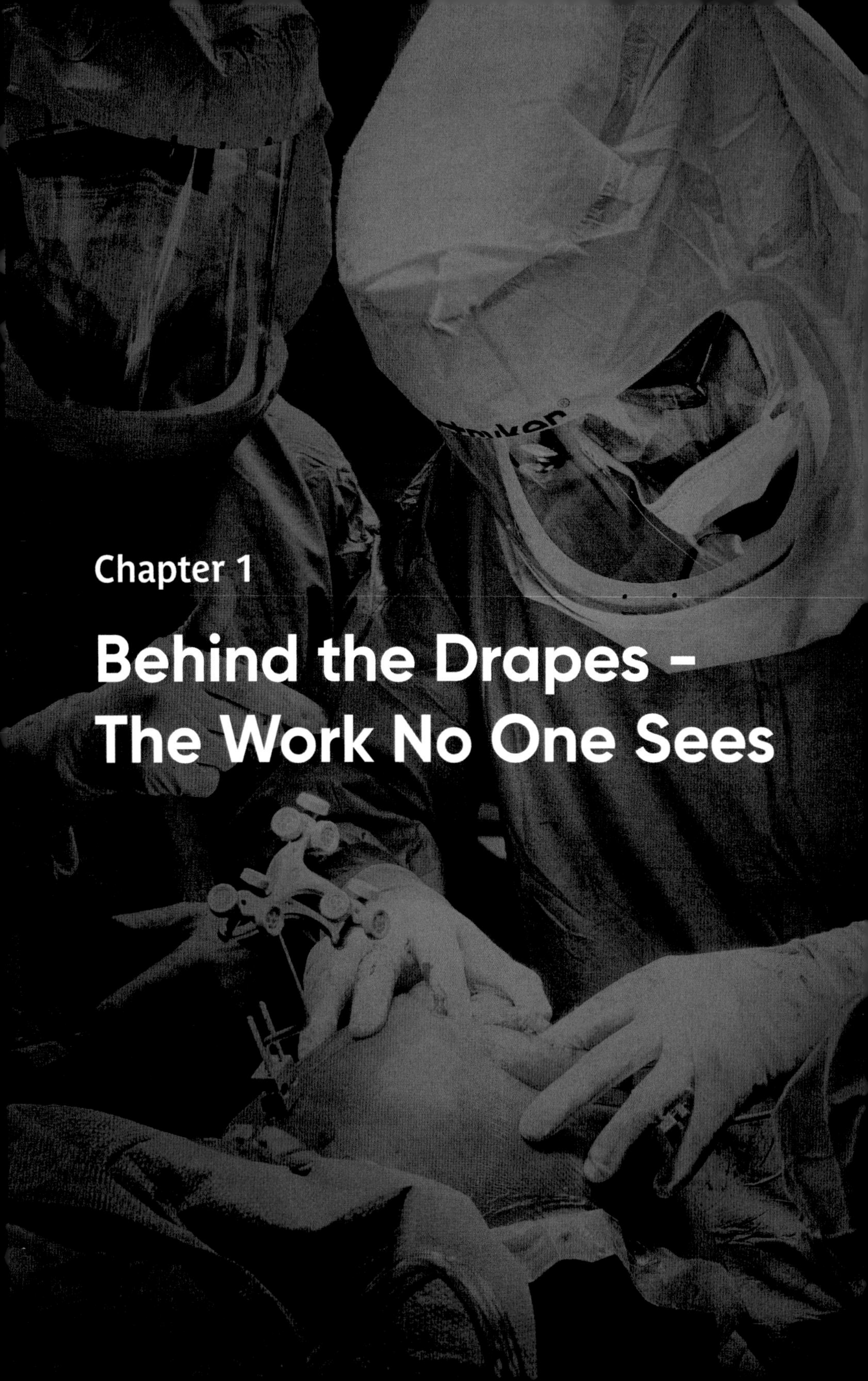

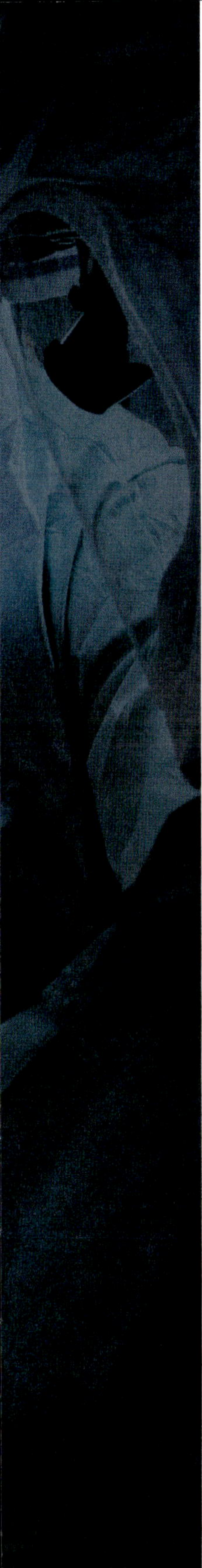

Once the drapes go up, and the operation starts, the anesthesiologist becomes invisible to most eyes. At least, that's how it looks to everyone else. From the outside, attention shifts to the surgical field. Lights focus where the incision will be made. Instruments line up neatly. Assistants focus on handing equipment to the surgeons. Conversations revolve around anatomy, surgical incision, exposure, and technique. The drama, if there is any, appears to live only one side of the surgical drapes.

On the other side at the head of the OR table, something deceivingly quieter happens. This is where anesthesiology lives. The patient is no longer talking. They cannot feel pain, and they cannot protect themselves, either. They cannot warn you when something feels wrong. Every safeguard that normally keeps a human alive: breathing, blood pressure regulation, temperature control, reflexes has been deliberately weakened or taken over by administering anesthesia. And for the duration of the operation, all of that responsibility belongs to you. It is a strange kind of intimacy. Brutally exposed.

You learn to know the patient without talking to them

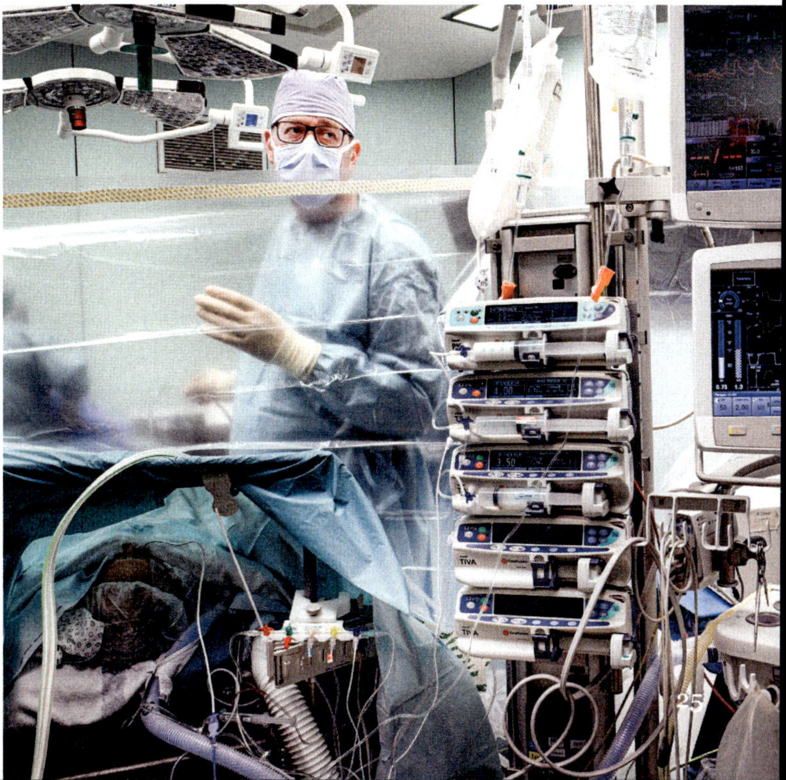

during their most vulnerable moments. A subtle drop in blood pressure tells you more than words ever could. A trend in breathing rate, a change in airway pressure speaks before lungs do.

A drifting end-tidal CO_2 curve may be the first hint of low cardiac output state, bleeding, dislodged a blood clot, or a failing heart. These signals arrive quietly, long before alarms may warn you that something is worth worrying about.

Fundamentally, anesthesiology is not reactive medicine, it is anticipatory. One of the most important trained virtues of an anesthesiologist is the ability to notice the trends in information displayed on the monitors, synthesizing the numbers with the experience and patterns learned, diagnosing the pathophysi-

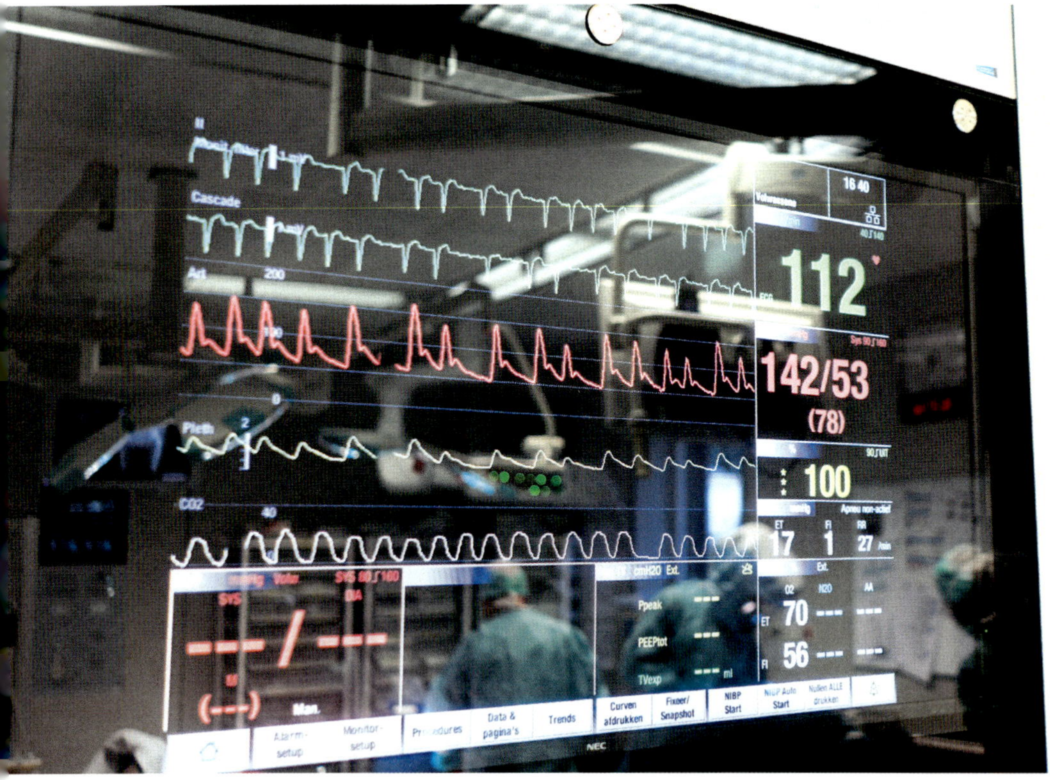

ologic processes and preventing further deterioration before reversing the down spiral.

When I stand between the head of the bed and maze of monitors and controls on an anesthesia machine, my eyes follow a pattern almost without thinking: quick glance over the information about the oxygen saturation, then exhaled carbon dioxide, CO_2. We are trained to understand that ventilation and circulation announce themselves there early, then the blood pressure trend, then the airway pressures and tidal volumes, then the rhythm on the ECG monitor... Anesthesiologists are not hunting for a single "warning number or parameter." They are uniquely trained to recognize a trend, an unfolding story that no one else in the operating room can see yet.

In fact, much of the anesthesiologist's work happens before anything goes wrong. Fluids are adjusted before hypotension becomes dangerous. Potent vascular constrictors (vasopressors) to correct dangerously low blood pressure, are given before blood supply heads dangerously south. Ventilation is fine tuned before lungs stiffen, atelectasis occurs, small airways start closing, or before oxygen in blood start going South. Pain pathways are blocked before the first surgical incision arrives.

If all of this is done well, no one actually notices. That is perhaps why some people who are not familiar with anesthesiology in many areas of the world call anesthesiologists "sleep doctors". Sometimes they say that anesthesia is boring once the patient is asleep. That nothing happens "in the middle." That the only important parts are "going to sleep and wake up", or the takeoff and landing.

That view has little to do with the reality. There is no autopilot in anesthesiology. The physiology is constantly tested by blood loss, by consequences of the body positioning for the operation, by surgical stress, by comorbid disease that doesn't read the textbook. Two patients undergoing the same operation can behave in entirely different ways. One tolerates everything effortlessly. The other unravels with the slightest provocation. Your job is to recognize which one you are dealing with; often before the difference becomes obvious.

Much of anesthesiologists' work is invisible because it is preventative by nature. Success in anesthesia is defined by the absence of complications. When things go right, nothing memorable happens. But when they go wrong, everything happens at once. And when that moment comes, there is no committee meeting. No pause button. Decisions are made in seconds, based on years of training and hundreds of similar moments stored somewhere in muscle memory and intuition. You learn to stay calm not because you don't feel pressure, but because panic wastes time-and time is physiology at risk.

It is also where the loneliness of the specialty reveals itself. You are always surrounded by people in the operating room, yet the responsibility for the patient's physiology rests squarely on your shoulders. The OR teams work together: Surgeons focus forward. Nurses manage flow of the surgical instruments. But the anesthesiologist watches everything

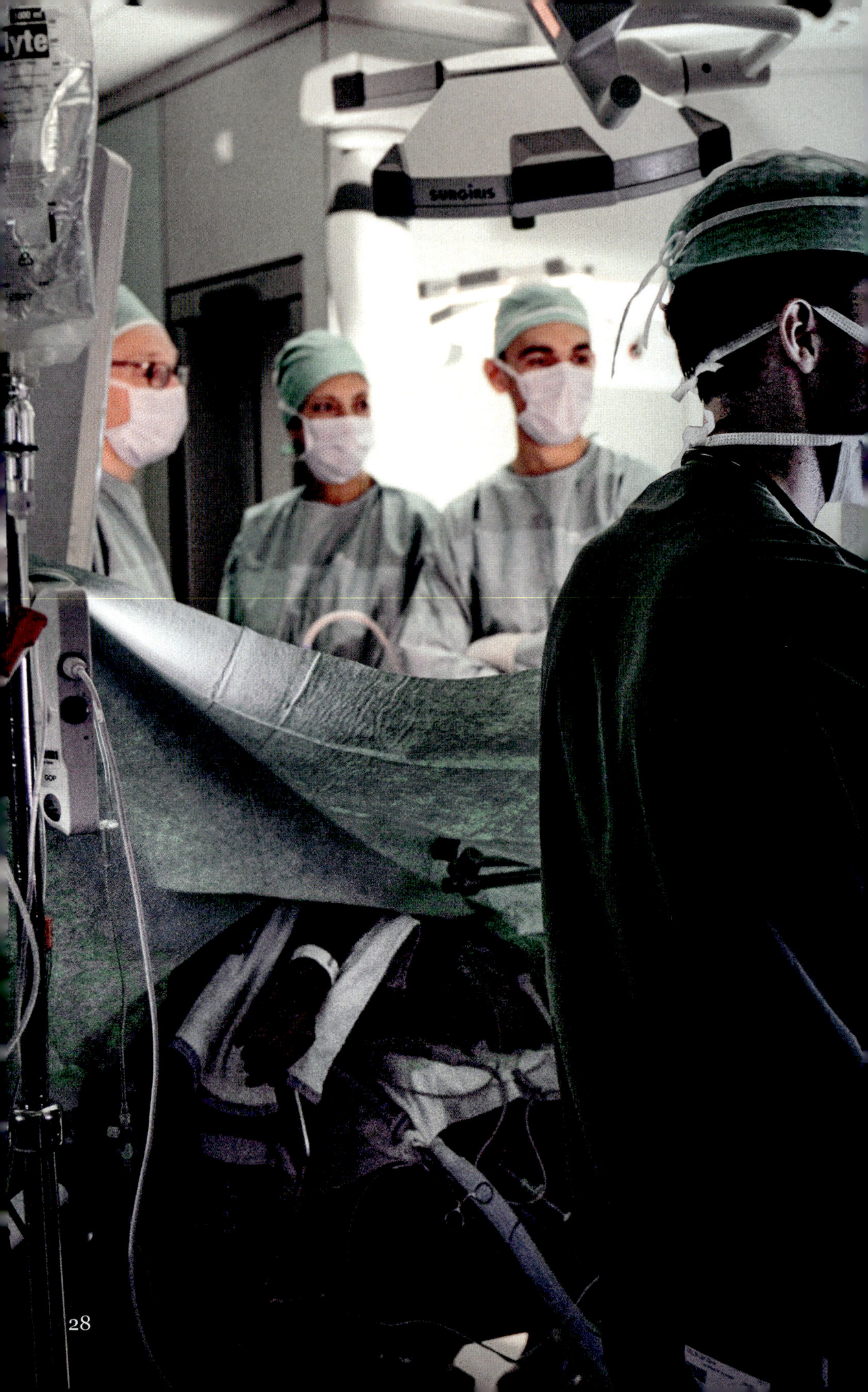
SURGIRIS

in solitude: patient, monitors, surgical rhythm, blood loss, medications, equipment, all while thinking several steps ahead. You are expected to be ready for complications that may never come, and held responsible if you weren't ready when they do.

There is no applause for what we do. There is only trust. Trust that the patient will wake up fine. Trust that organs were protected. Trust that pain will be controlled. Trust that the invisible work mattered. When the case ends and the surgical drapes come down, the patient returns to view. If all went well, they breathe, open their eyes, and are wheeled away to the recovery room. The room resets. The monitors quiet down. The maze is dismantled. And once again, it looks like nothing happened. But at the head of the table, everything did.

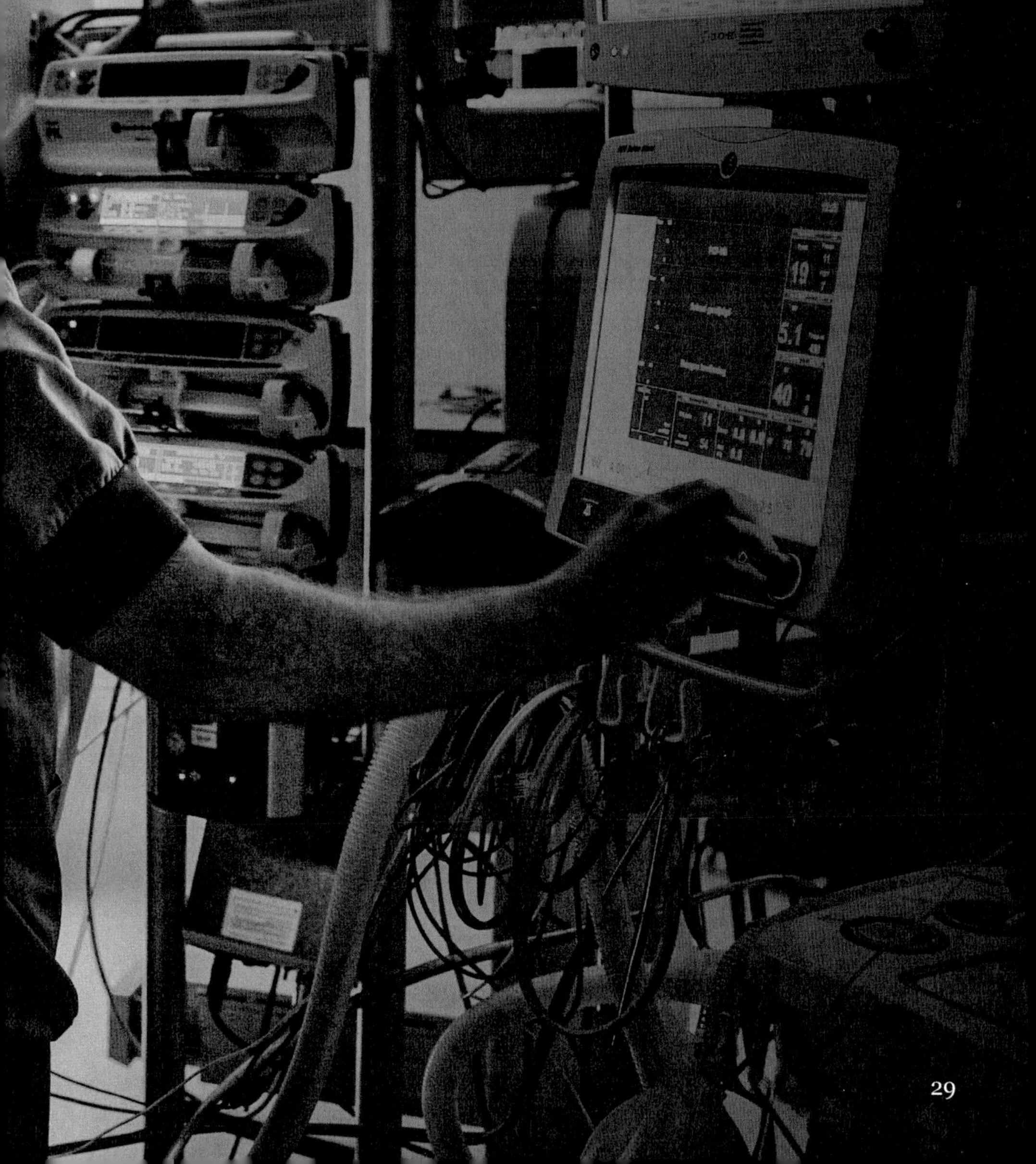

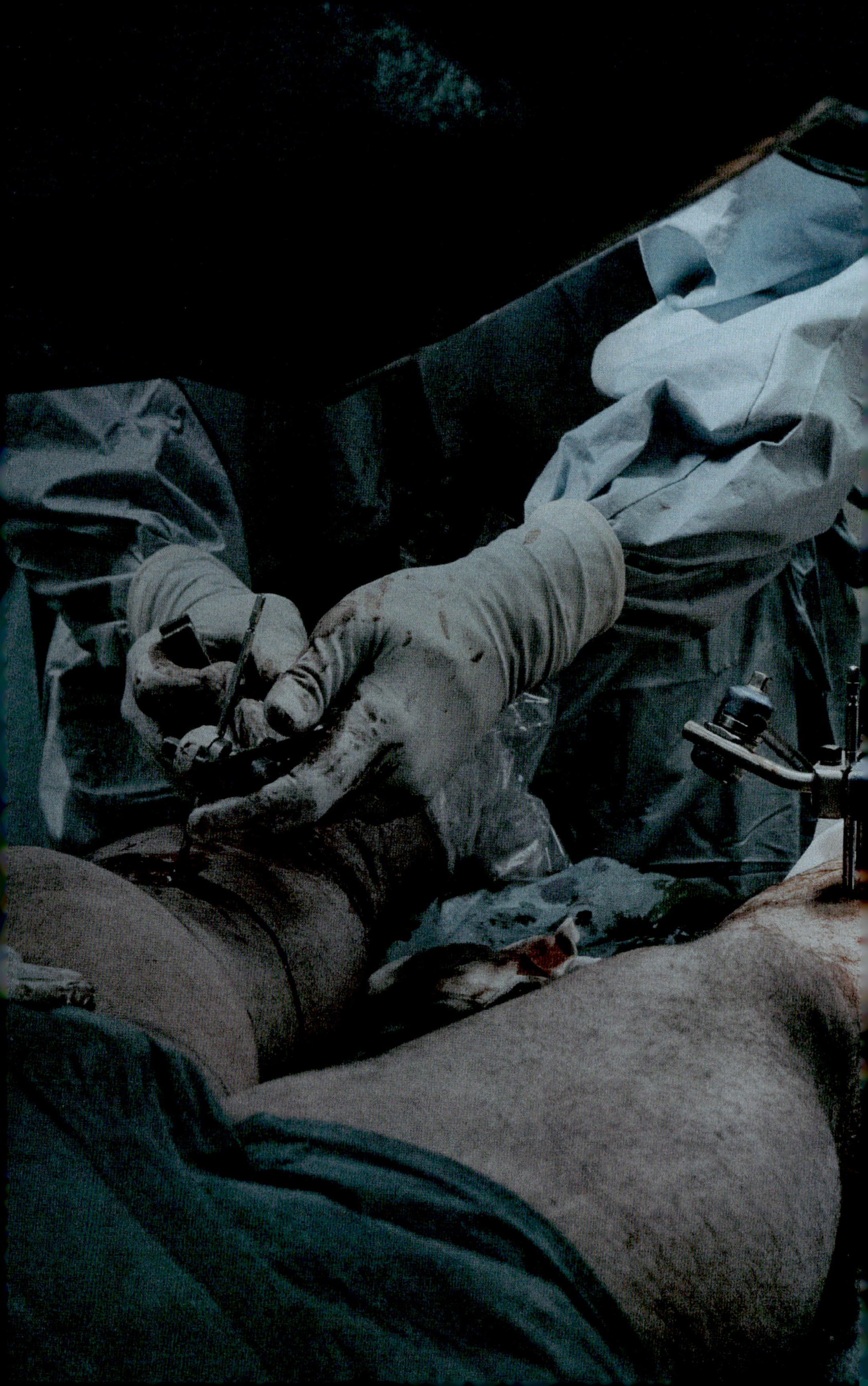

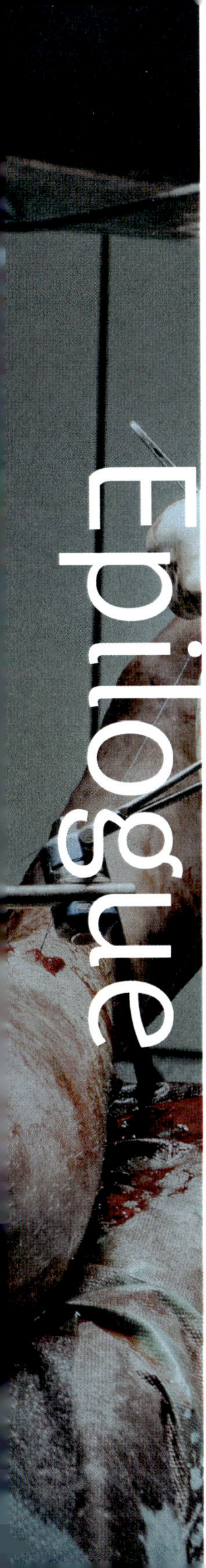

A Heartbeat Continues

After years in trauma rooms - from New York to Europe I learned how little margin there often is. A case can shift from stable to unstable in minutes. Blood loss, airway difficulty, a heart that does not behave as expected. What matters is not the drama of the moment, but whether the

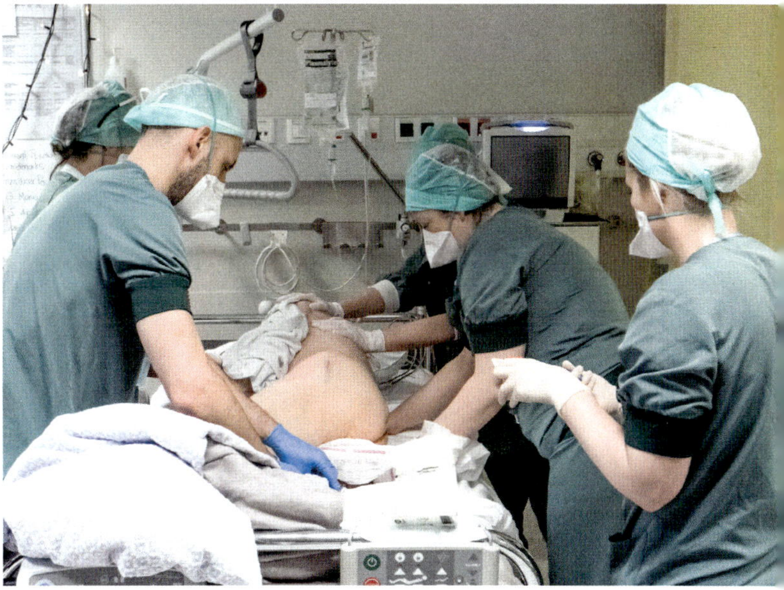

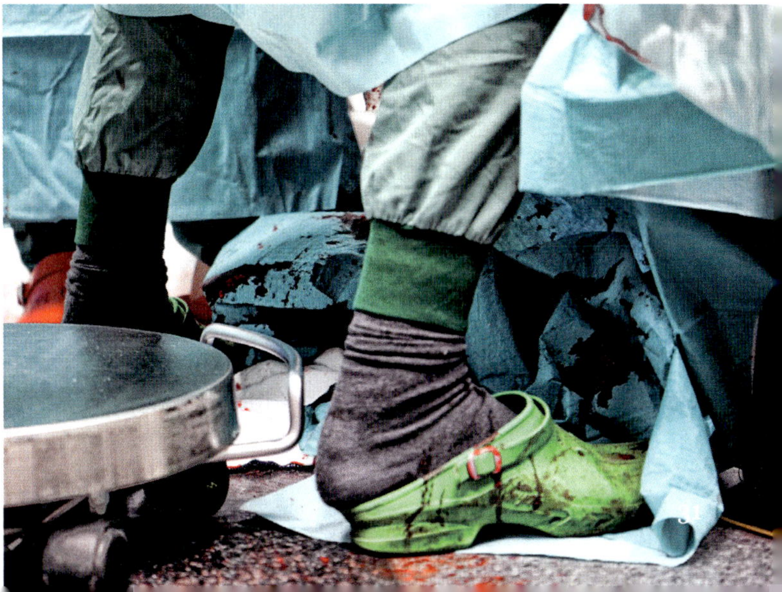

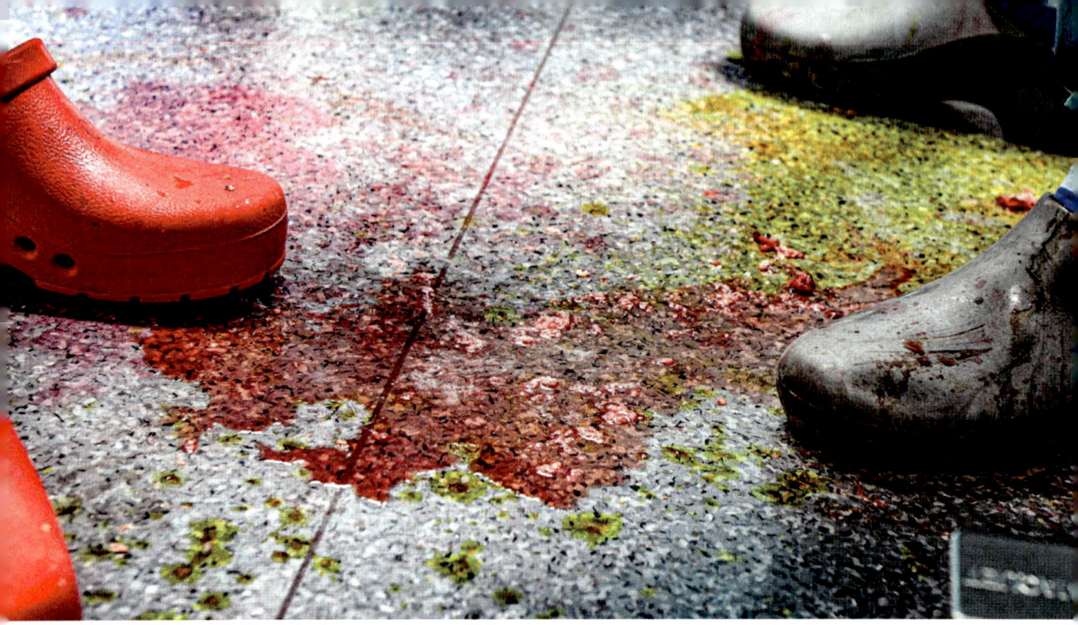

change is recognized early enough to correct and reverse it.

This is where anesthesiology lives. Not in chaos, and not in calm, but in the narrow space where physiology is continuously managed and protected. Surgeons repair what is visible. Anesthesiologists anticipate what comes next, they hold the life line, assure oxygen delivery to the essential organs, circulation, and time. That work rarely announces itself. When it succeeds, it looks like nothing happened. When it fails, it becomes impossible to ignore.

We work in that space every day. Not occasionally. That is our routine responsibility.

Being an anesthesiologist is not for everyone. You cannot do this work without learning something about uncertainty and restraint. You see tragedy and randomness, but also

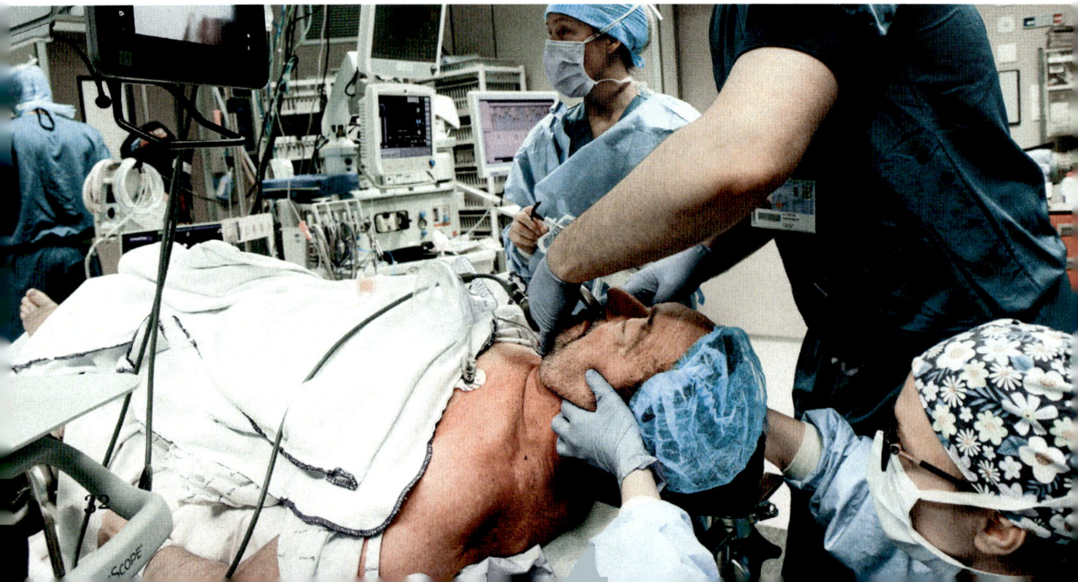

resilience and recovery. You learn how quickly conditions change, and how little warning you are given when they do. Over time, you learn to stay calm when others cannot.

What changes over time is your relationship with the responsibility. You stop seeking recognition and start valuing reliability, endurance and diligence. You learn and accept that success in anesthesiology is often invisible, and that the best days are the ones where nothing remarkable happens.

A patient wakes up. Breathing on their own. Unaware of how close physiology may have come to its limits. That is enough.

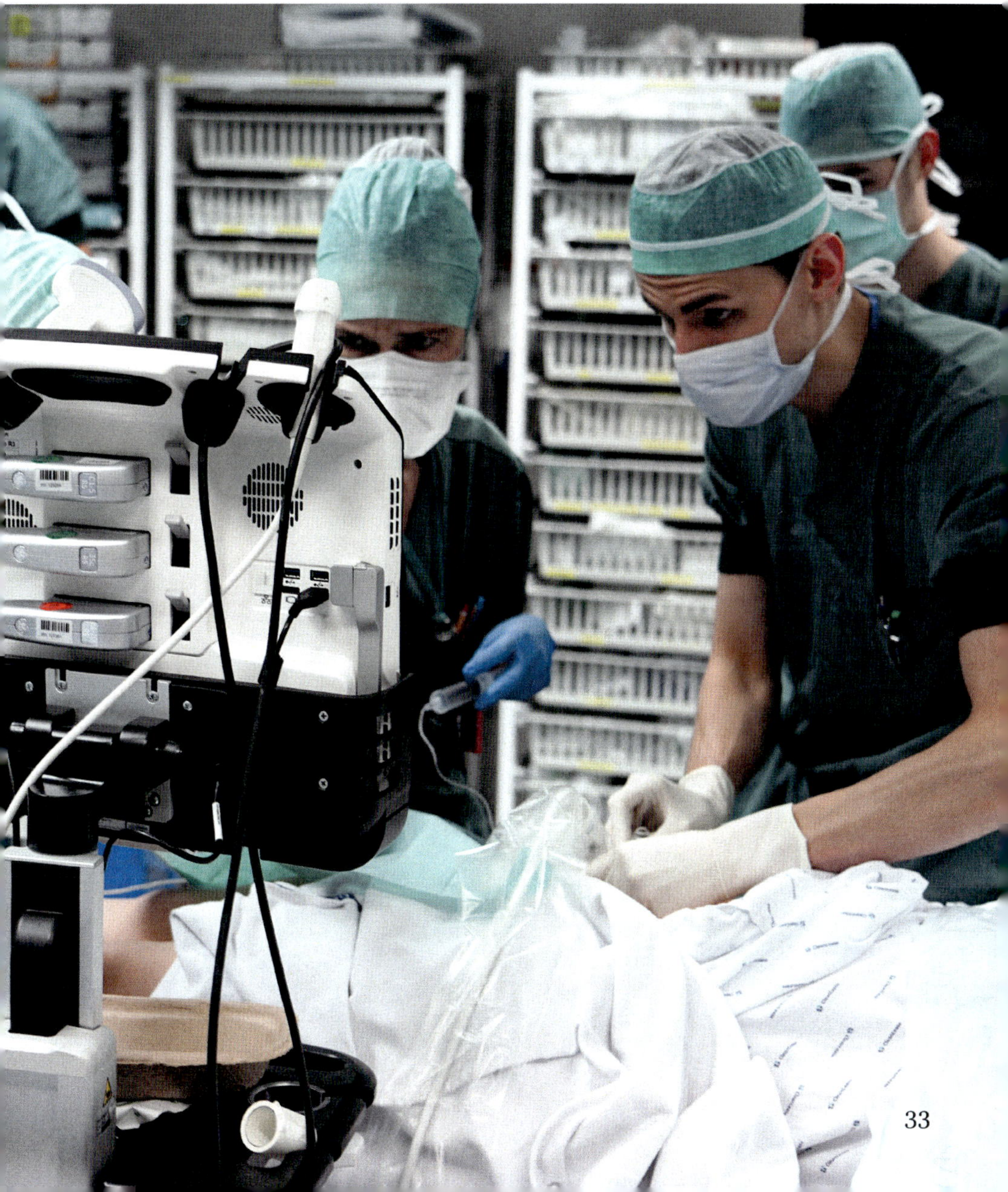

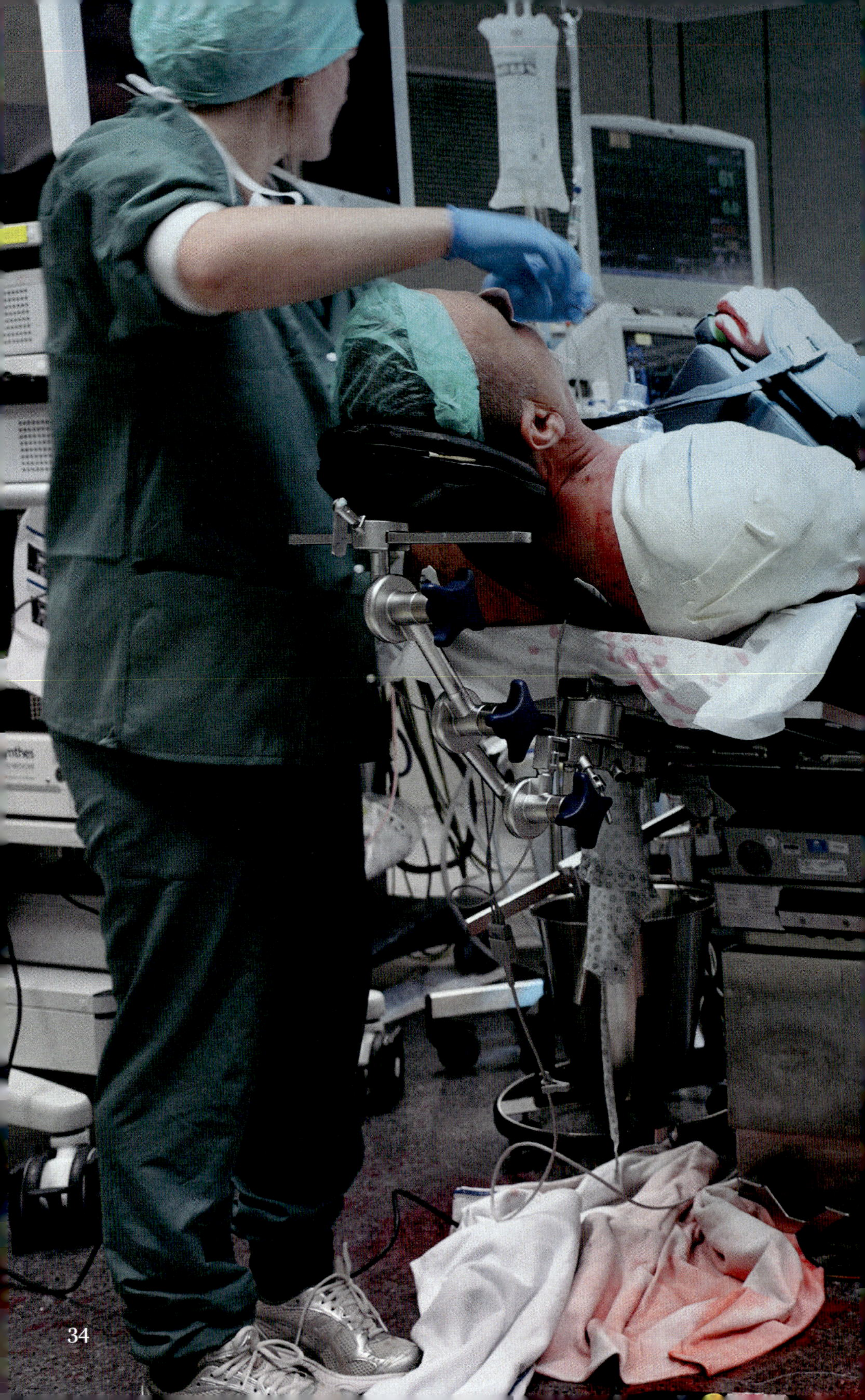

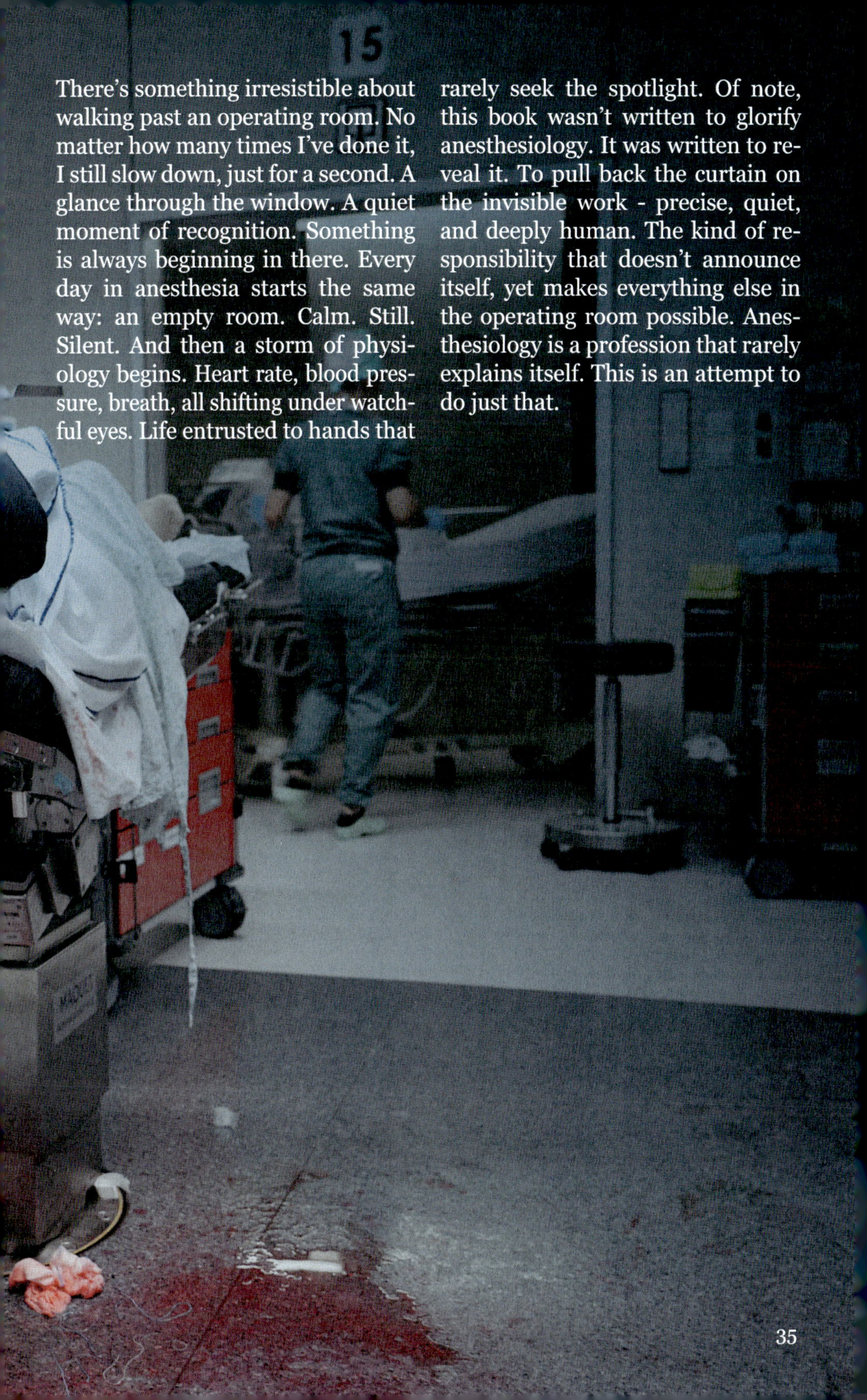

There's something irresistible about walking past an operating room. No matter how many times I've done it, I still slow down, just for a second. A glance through the window. A quiet moment of recognition. Something is always beginning in there. Every day in anesthesia starts the same way: an empty room. Calm. Still. Silent. And then a storm of physiology begins. Heart rate, blood pressure, breath, all shifting under watchful eyes. Life entrusted to hands that rarely seek the spotlight. Of note, this book wasn't written to glorify anesthesiology. It was written to reveal it. To pull back the curtain on the invisible work - precise, quiet, and deeply human. The kind of responsibility that doesn't announce itself, yet makes everything else in the operating room possible. Anesthesiology is a profession that rarely explains itself. This is an attempt to do just that.

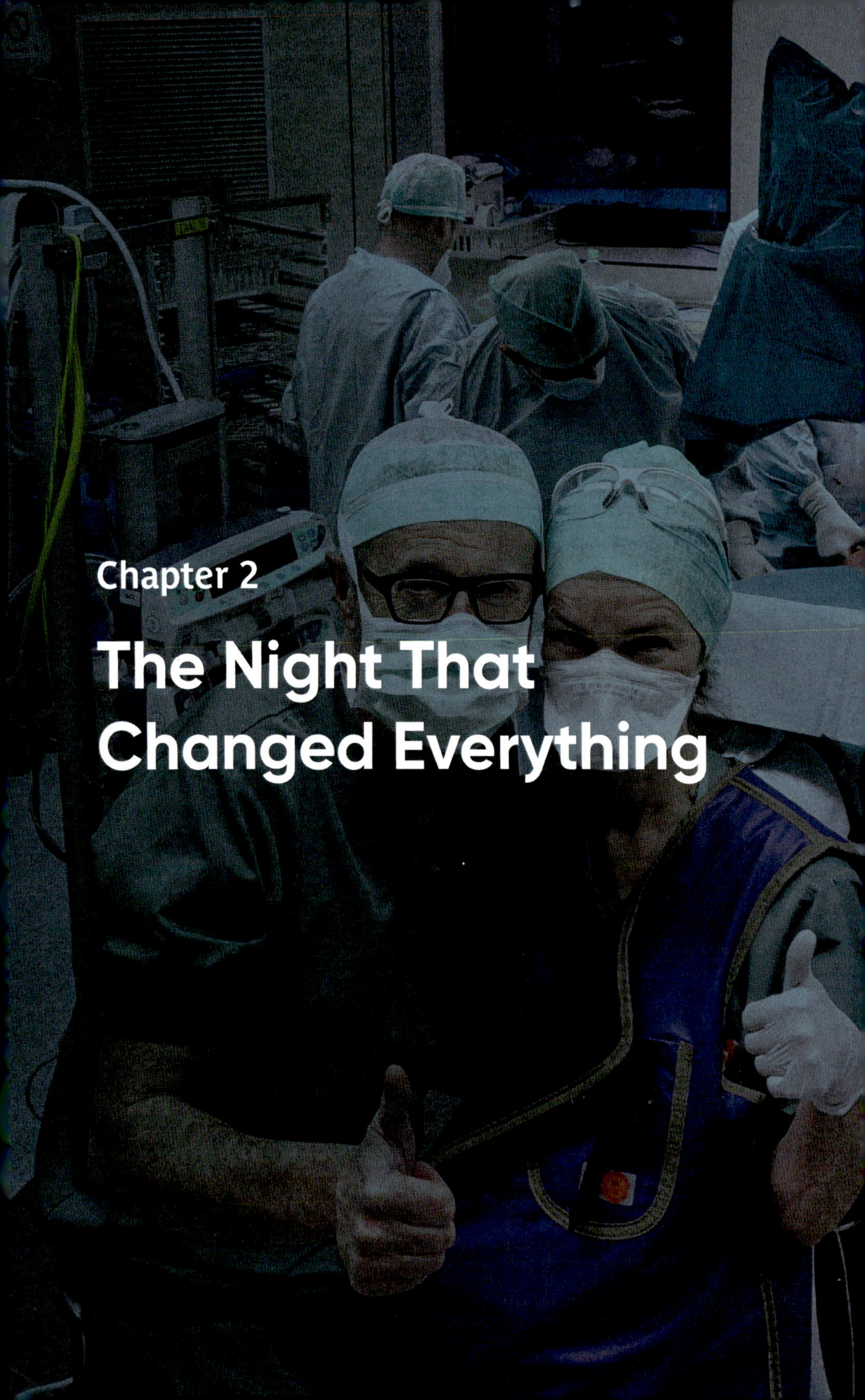

Chapter 2

The Night That Changed Everything

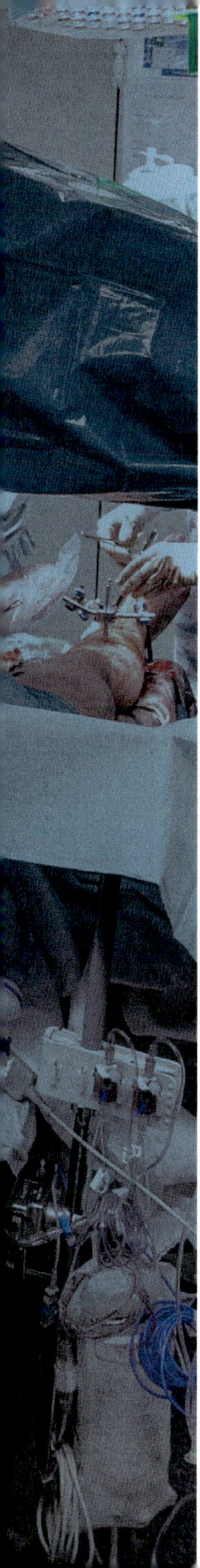

Early on in my career, I did not fully understand what anesthesiologists actually do, like most people, and event many doctors. Anesthesiologists work largely out of sight, in operating rooms and in intensive care units. They live a professional life that intersects with everyone else's, yet it is rarely fully seen to actually grasp what they do.

Early in my medical training, I imagined a different future. I was an internal medicine resident, drawn toward cardiology and electrophysiology, hoping to unite my love of medicine with a lifelong fascination for electronics. Since my teenage years, I have spent countless hours playing music, building instruments, amplifiers, and loudspeakers, and working in recording studios as a sound engineer. I worried that a career in medicine might sever that connection, that full immersion would leave no room for the creative, technical world that had shaped me. Electrophysiology seemed like the perfect compromise: intellectually rigorous, technologically driven, and focused on pacemakers, defibrillators, and the elegant logic of electric cardiac circuits. It felt like a path that could preserve both identities. Then one night, everything changed.

I was on night duty as a Chief resident at St. Joseph's Medical Center in Paterson, New Jersey. It was the 1990s, at the height of the AIDS epidemic. As a senior resident, I covered the Critical Care Unit, patient admissions through the emergency department, and emergency calls throughout the hospital. Late that evening, a STAT call came from the cardiology ward, the post-cardiac catheterization unit, where one of the patients was in dire straits. I ran upstairs to the 4th floor with two junior residents.

The scene was chaotic. A man in his sixties lay pulseless, blue, and motionless. Nurses struggled to obtain IV access through collapsed, overused veins. The respiratory therapist attempted to help him breath via a bag-mask, but his cheeks merely ballooned; air was going in, yet none was reaching the lungs. We all rotated through chest compressions, uncomfortably aware that without an airway, breathing and access to the circulation, we were losing him.

This was in the early 1990's before the era of modern digital monitoring. The ECG was a continuous paper rhythm strip, crawling steadily out of the ECG machine, showing pulseless electrical activity. We analyzed the tracing, debated the rhythm, and discussed the physiology in detail, armed with knowledge, terminology, and theory, while the patient, deprived of oxygen and circulation, continued to slip away. What we lacked, painfully and unmistakably, were the fundamental, technical skills that actually save lives.

Then voices from the hallway cut through the noise.

"*Excuse us! Excuse us!*"

The anesthesiology team that routinely responded to resuscitations just arrived.

A senior anesthesiologist and his anesthesiology student moved straight to the head of the bed. They asked a few precise questions; no hesitation, no commentary, and immediately took control of the airway. Within seconds, the breathing tube was in place. Oxygenation followed. Color returned. Calm, authoritative instructions replaced the confusion. Chest compressions became effective. Circulation began to reappear.

They asked if we needed help with intravenous access. We sure did.

In just a couple of minutes, the anesthesiology team placed a large-bore central line in the right internal jugular vein. With reliable access to the central circulation, resuscitation medications were administered. Seconds later, the ECG rhythm corrected. Blood pressure returned.

Life resumed. And just as quietly as they had arrived, the anesthesiologists left. They asked if we needed any other help. When we said no, they returned to their tasks, somewhere in the vaults of the operating room.

The patient lived.

I finished my night shift without having fully processed what I had just witnessed. But driving home next morning, alone in the quiet, it settled in with unexpected force. Despite all our internal medicine medical knowledge, despite understanding the physiology and the theory in detail, we had not possessed the skills that were needed to save that patient's life. The anesthesiologists did.

That realization stayed with me. I wanted those skills. I wanted to be able to act when seconds mattered, not just explain what was happening, but change the outcome. I understood then that no matter how much I loved the internal medicine, I would never feel complete practicing medicine without that life-savers ability.

That week I changed course.

I walked away from internal medicine training and prestigious cardiology fellowship that I had lined up at St. Joseph's and began residency in anesthesiology at St. Luke's-Roosevelt Hospital in New York. It remains one of the best professional decisions I have ever made. Looking back now, after three decades in the OR at the head of the bed, I know what moved me that night. It was competence under pressure. The confidence to take over when the body fails.

That is why I became an anesthesiologist.

Not for recognition.

But to be useful when life is on the line. And to step away quietly when it isn't.

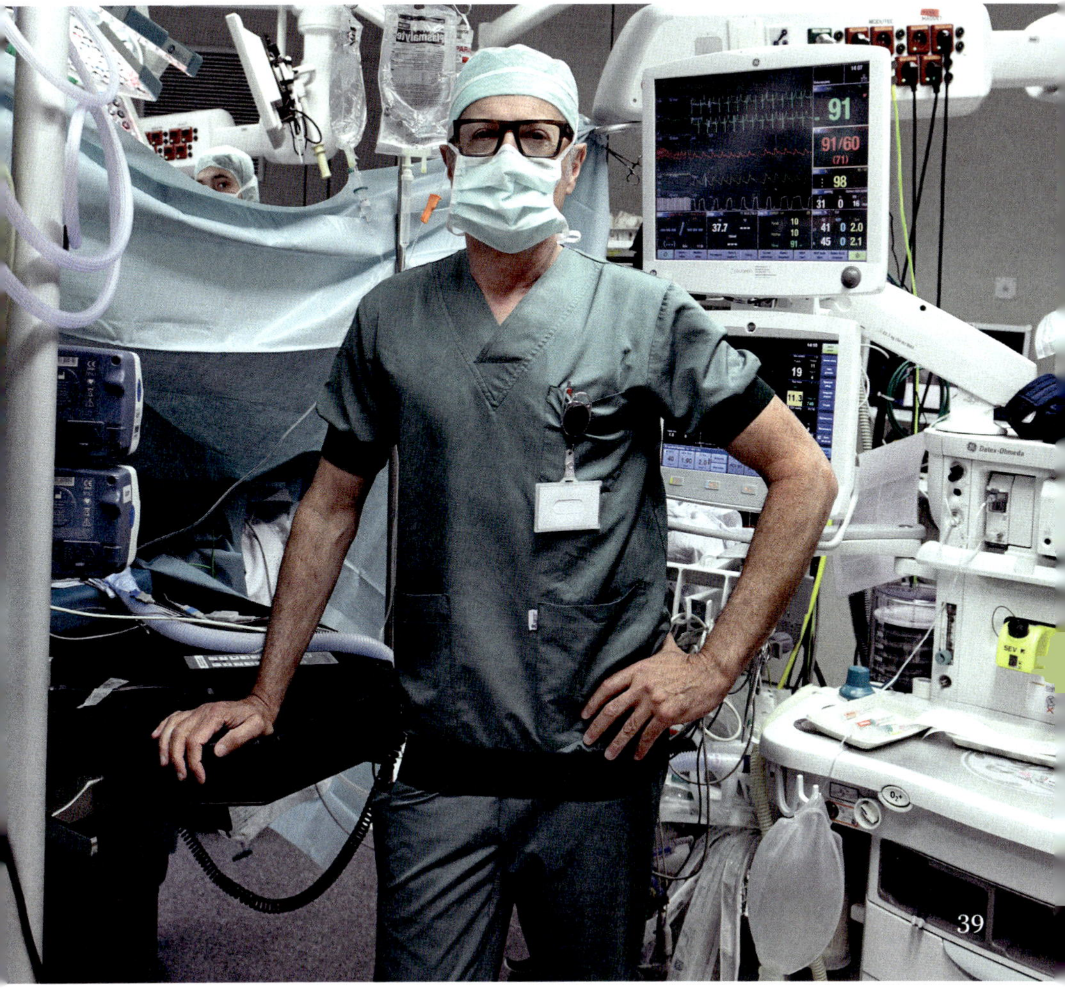

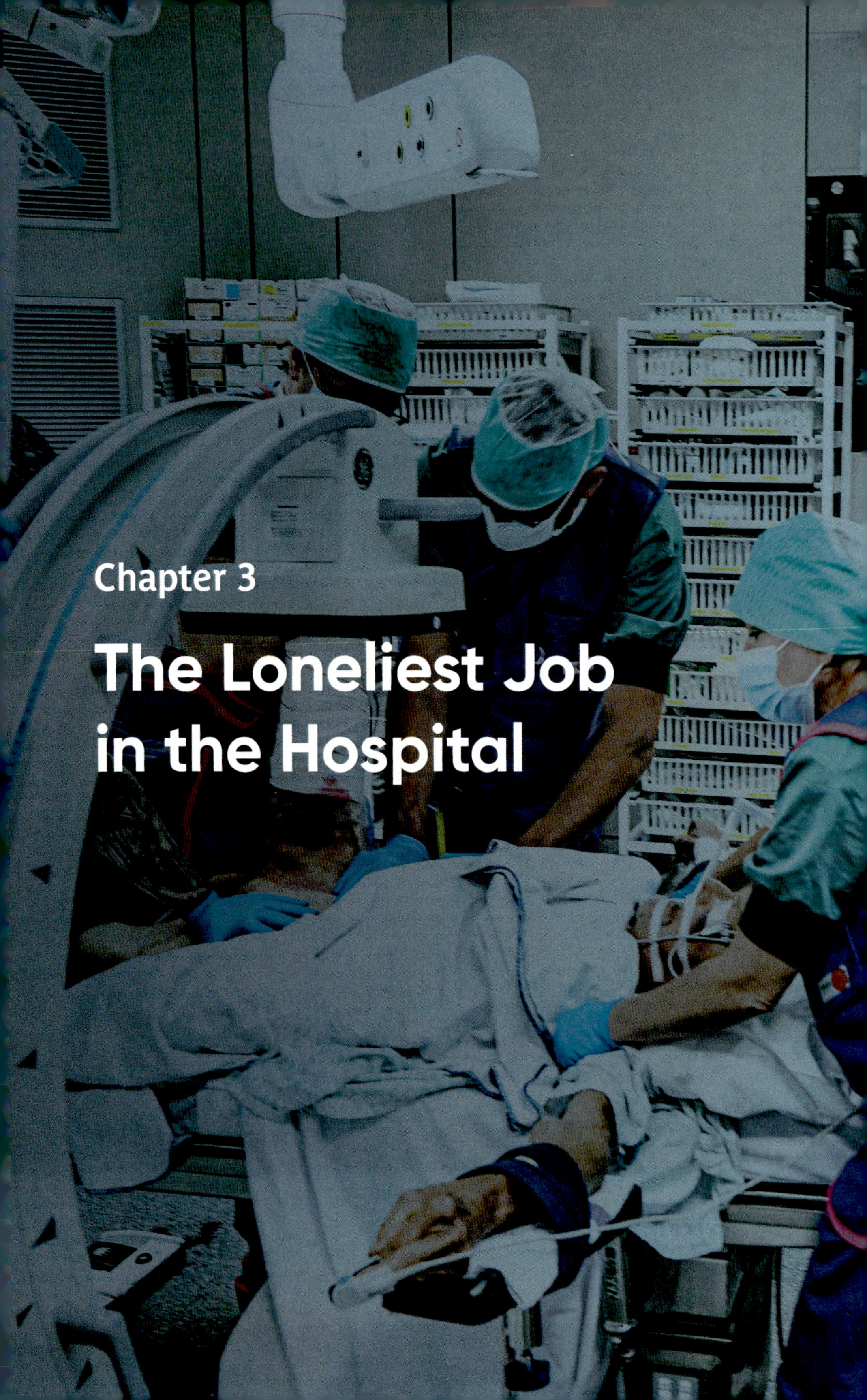

Chapter 3

The Loneliest Job in the Hospital

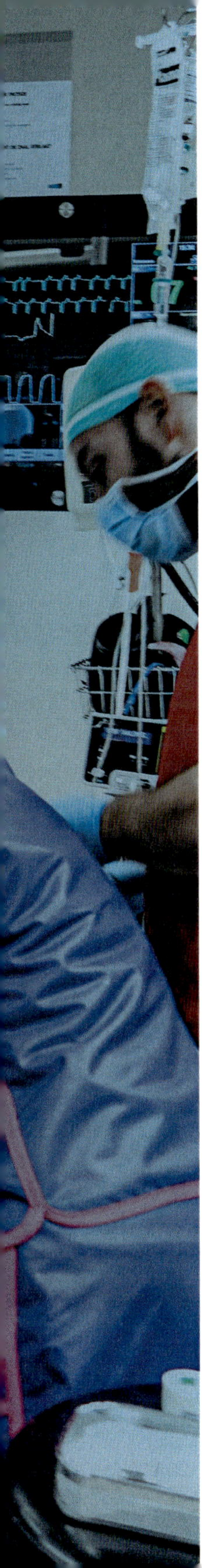

Christmas, Thanksgiving, and New Years are meant for family. They are supposed to be filled with shared meals, familiar voices, children staying up too late, and the comfort of being together. For most people, the idea of working through these nights feels almost unthinkable. For anesthesiologists and for surgeons, nurses, and hospital staff, it is routine.

While the world slows down, hospitals do not. While cities celebrate, operating rooms remain lit. Somewhere, behind closed doors and drawn curtains, physiology still needs help. Trauma still arrives. Emergencies do not check the calendar.

There is a particular quiet to the hospital at night. Hallways feel longer. Footsteps echo in empty corridors. The operating room in the dark looks somewhat like an airplane cockpit suspended in space. Monitors hum softly, a galore of small LED lights across anesthesia machine and multiple monitors mounted on top of it. Infusion pumps lights blink away in stand-by mode. Outside, people chant, they watch fireworks. Inside, you watch waveforms on the cardiovascular and respiratory monitors.

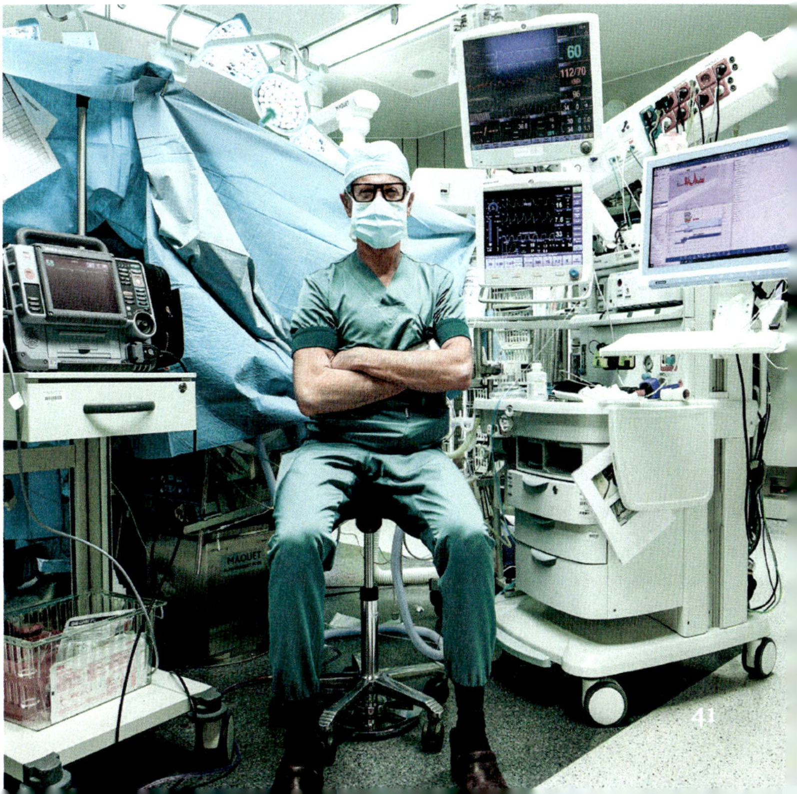

I remember many mornings finishing a trauma case and watching the sun rise over Spanish Harlem, the New York City slowly reawakening in front of me. I would wonder how other people had lived through the night: where they had been, what their hours had held and how different it must feel to wake up rested, to step into the early morning light ready for a new day.As I made my way home, I carried a different kind of fatigue. Not just physical tiredness, but the heavy weight that comes from witnessing intense human tragedies that most people never see. The hallways at St. Luke's Hospital, at 114th Street and Amsterdam Avenue, were still active, still busy, even as the world outside moved on quietly toward breakfast and morning routines. I have worked enough nights, and holidays, to recognize the feeling before I even enter the operating room: the building where you work remains fully awake, while life beyond its walls continues without you.

Sometimes it's a small moment that makes it real. A nurse hastily unwrapping sterile supplies while "Jingle Bells" leaks faintly from a phone somewhere down the corridor. A text message you read with gloved hands. A quick glance at a family photo as you pass the locker, just long enough to remember what you're missing, not long enough to dwell on it.

This is where anesthesiology reveals one of its less discussed truths: it can be profoundly solitary. Even in a busy operating room, much of your work happens in isolation. Decisions are internal. Judgments are silent. You may exchange words with the OR staff, but the responsibility to diagnose, to anticipate, to intervene, to act rests squarely with you. There is no one else at the head of the bed; you are the sole decision maker. The responsible captain of the ship.

On the night shift ("night call"), the contrast sharpens. You can feel celebration of the life in the air outside the hospital; distant, unreal, while inside you are doing the oldest thing medicine does: guarding breath and circulation.

When I mentor students considering medicine, I tell them this early: medicine is not a job: It is a way of living. Failing to understand this leads inevitably to frustration, resentment, unhappiness, or burnout.

Anesthesiology reflects this reality more than most fields of medicine. You leave home before others wake and return after the lights are off. You miss dinners. You miss birthdays. You learn how often you must explain, sometimes to your family, sometimes to yourself, why you were not there.Over time, you adapt. You learn to focus completely when it matters, and to let go when you can.

If you were not an anesthesiologist, it would be difficult to fully grasp the weight of this role. Inside a maze of cables, monitors, and pathophysiology, anesthesiologists manage life

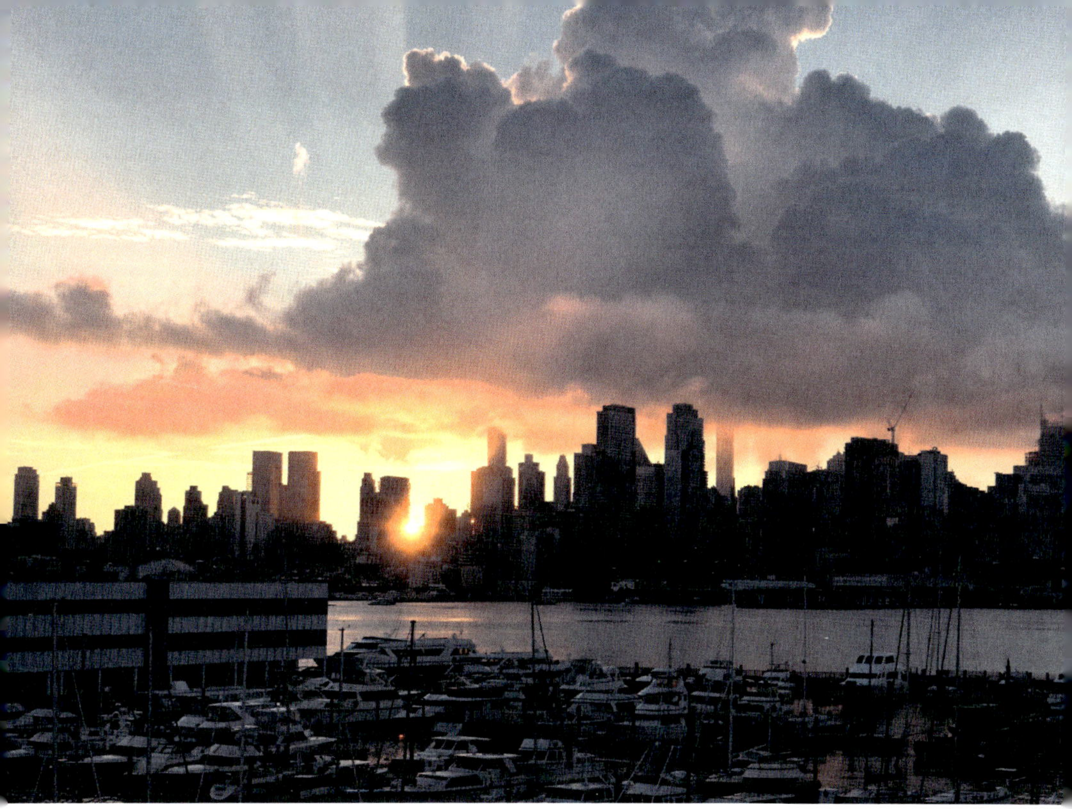

moment by moment. Anticipating instability before it becomes visible. Correcting dangerous twists of physiology before anyone else senses them. Making decisions that determine whether a patient safely passes through moments they could not survive otherwise.

The returning paradox is that when everything goes well, no one notices. There is no visible incision to admire. No before and after photograph. No obvious marker of success; except that the patient wakes up, intact, unaware of how close physiology may have drifted toward disaster. This invisibility can be isolating.

Yet there is also something grounding about it. In the quiet of the operating room, far from celebration and noise, anesthesiologists develop a deep respect for responsibility. You learn that meaning does not come from recognition, but from reliability. From being the constant presence when others rotate in and out. From knowing that while the world pauses for holidays, someone still has to keep the heart beating. And when you walk out of the hospital in the early hours of the morning, tired but steady, there is a particular kind of satisfaction in knowing that life continued. Because you were there.

Tomorrow, the room will be empty again. Calm. Silent.

And when it fills, you will be rested and ready to do the unseen work again.

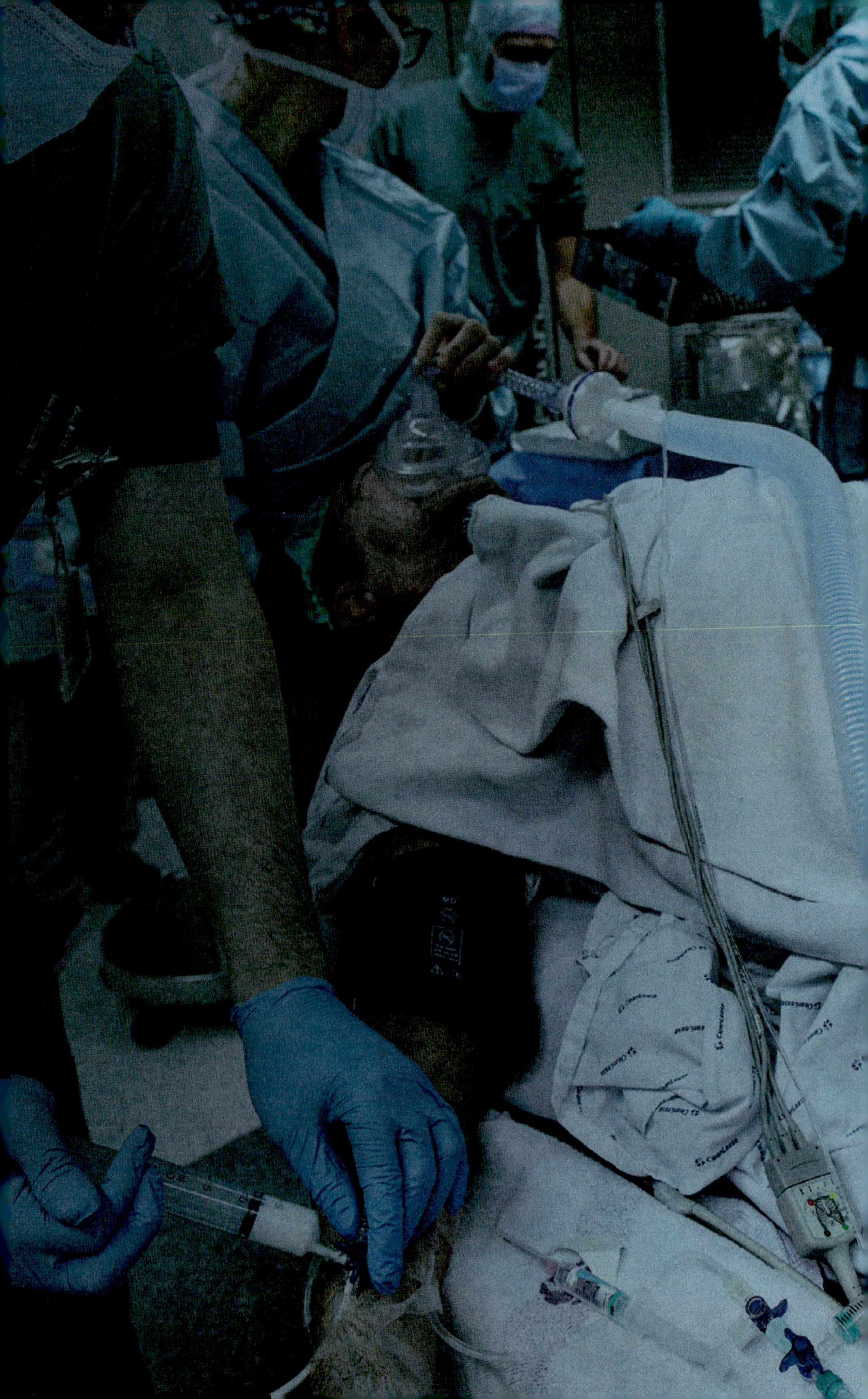

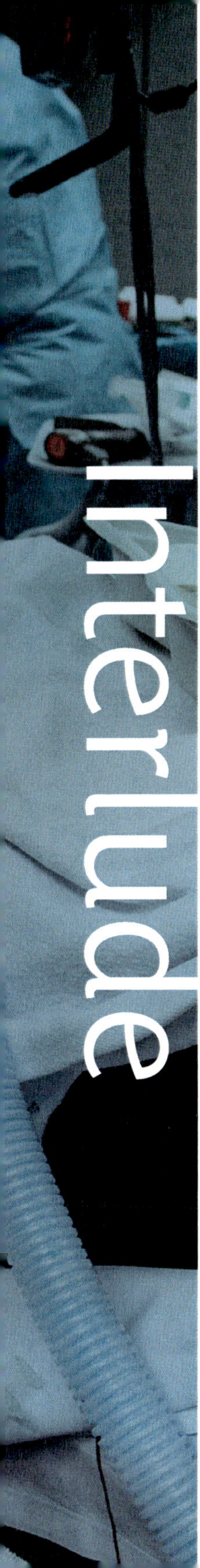

The Quiet Moment Before Everything Begins

There is a silent, profound moment in every anesthetic that few people notice. It happens just before induction; after the check lists, after the questions, after the monitors are connected. The room is not silent, it is buzzing with preparatory activity, but calm in a strange, recognizable way. The patient is still awake. The team is ready. Everything that can be prepared has been prepared.

The oxygen mask is close to patient's face ready to preoxygenate before the anesthesia induction. The syringes with anesthetics are drawn up, but not yet injected. You glance once more at the monitors.

In that instant, you always do the same quick scan: the oxygen saturation, end-tidal CO_2 line ready to write its first sentence, the blood pressure cycling, the ECG rhythm steady. Then you look back to the patient's face: skin tone, expression, small changes in muscle tension, details that, in this moment, matter more than the numbers on the screen.

The patient may look at you with the last grasp of consciousness. Sometimes they say nothing. Sometimes they ask a final question. Sometimes they try to make a joke. Sometimes they are afraid and don't know how to say it. And then there is the few seconds that last longer than it should: the quiet pause where you decide how to meet that fear.

Not with speeches. With presence. You might adjust the pillow, smooth the blanket, reposition the pulse oximeter that's pinching. You might place a hand on the patient's shoulder through the thin barrier of a gown and a warm forced air blanket, and say the simplest true sentence you have: "I'm right here. we've got you."

And in that moment, everything slows down.

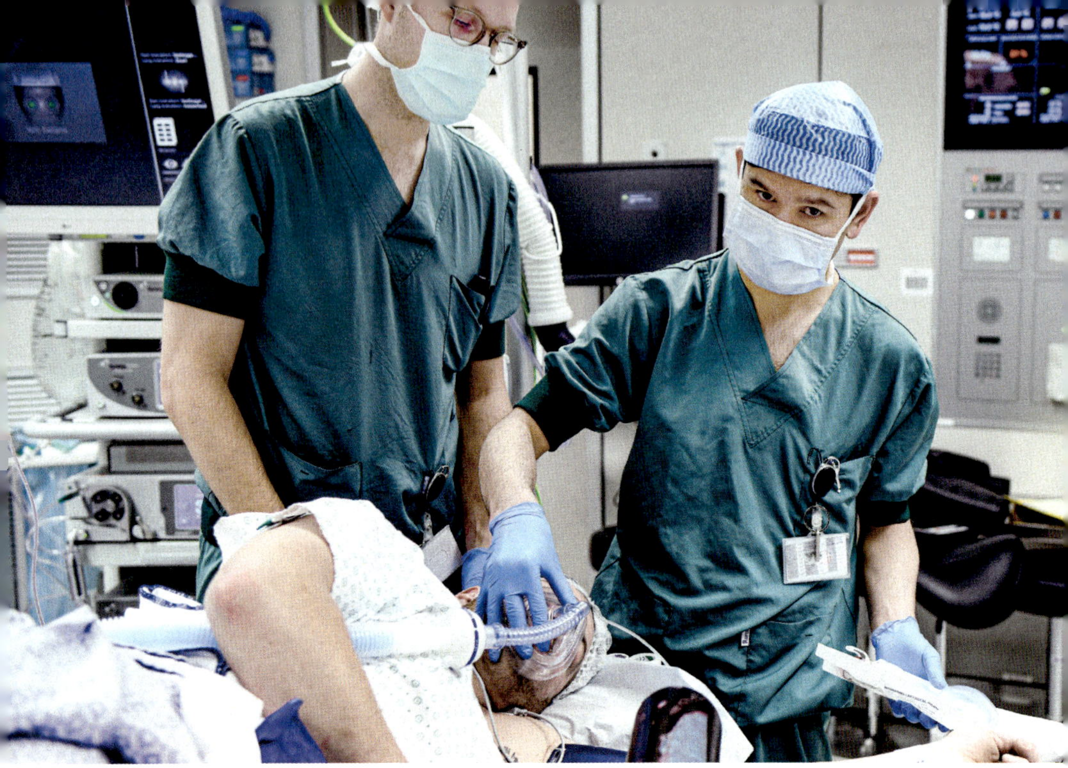

What happens next will separate the patient from consciousness, from pain, from control. For a short while, they will entrust their breathing, their circulation, and their safety to someone they may have met only minutes ago. At this point, there is no pause button.

That kind of trust is rare in life. It cannot be rushed. It cannot be automated. And it cannot be replaced by technology. This is why anesthesiology has always been uncomfortable with the idea of AI and automation replacing humans in this process.

Over the years, I have become convinced that technology does not belong in this moment. Not because technology is useless, but because this moment demands restraint. The tools that matter are the ones that quietly support, reinforce, and disappear into the background. Technology should assist routine decisions. It should strengthen memory, not replace thinking. It should never compete for attention when attention is life on the operating room table in front of you.

This is why thoughtful tools matter, and why complicated ones do not. Because when the patient's eyes close, when the breathing start to cease, when physiology begins to drift, there is no algorithm that will feel the weight of that responsibility.

Only you. And when the induction and the operation begin, when the storm arrives, this quiet moment will already have done its work for the smooth course during the operation.

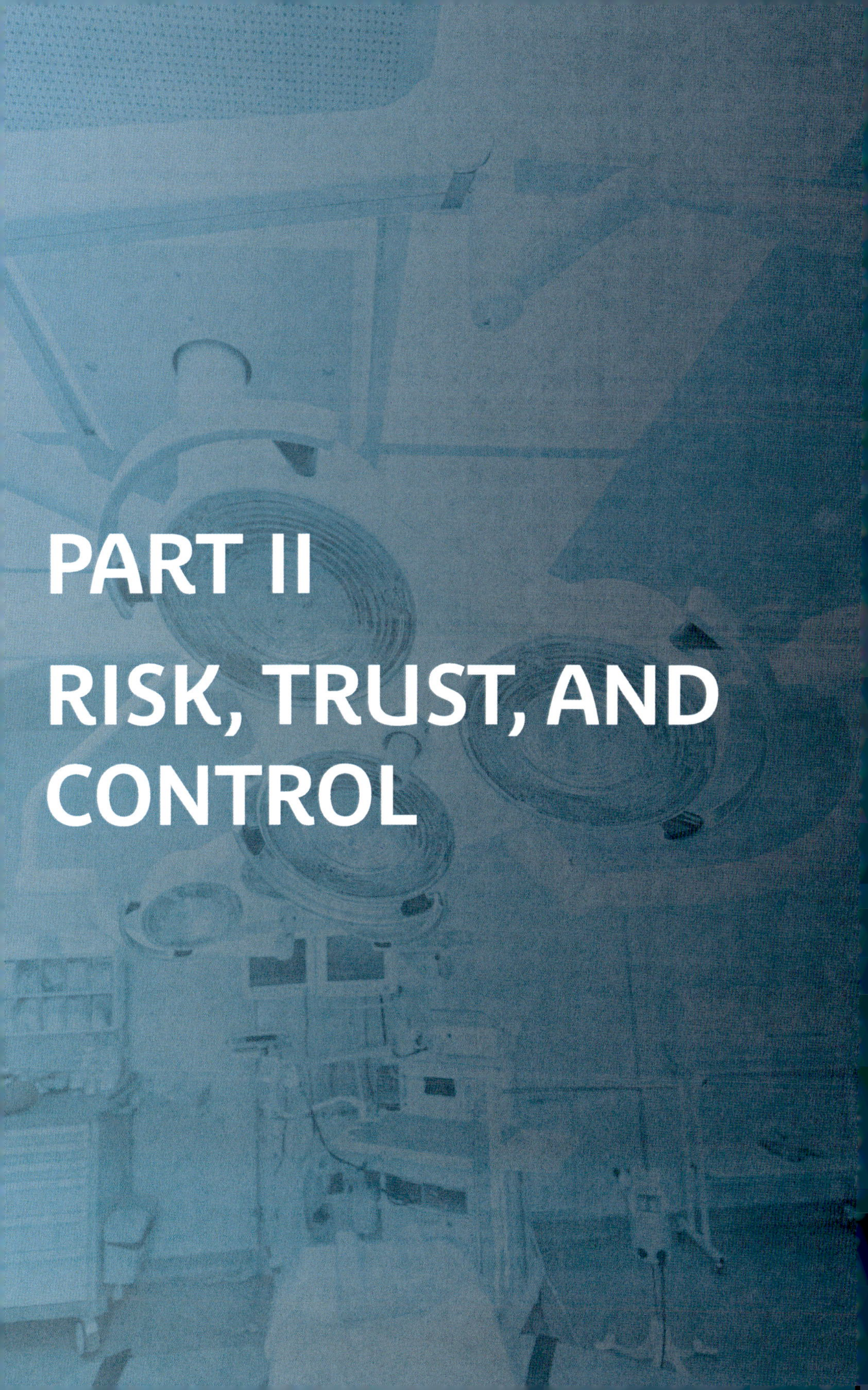

PART II

RISK, TRUST, AND CONTROL

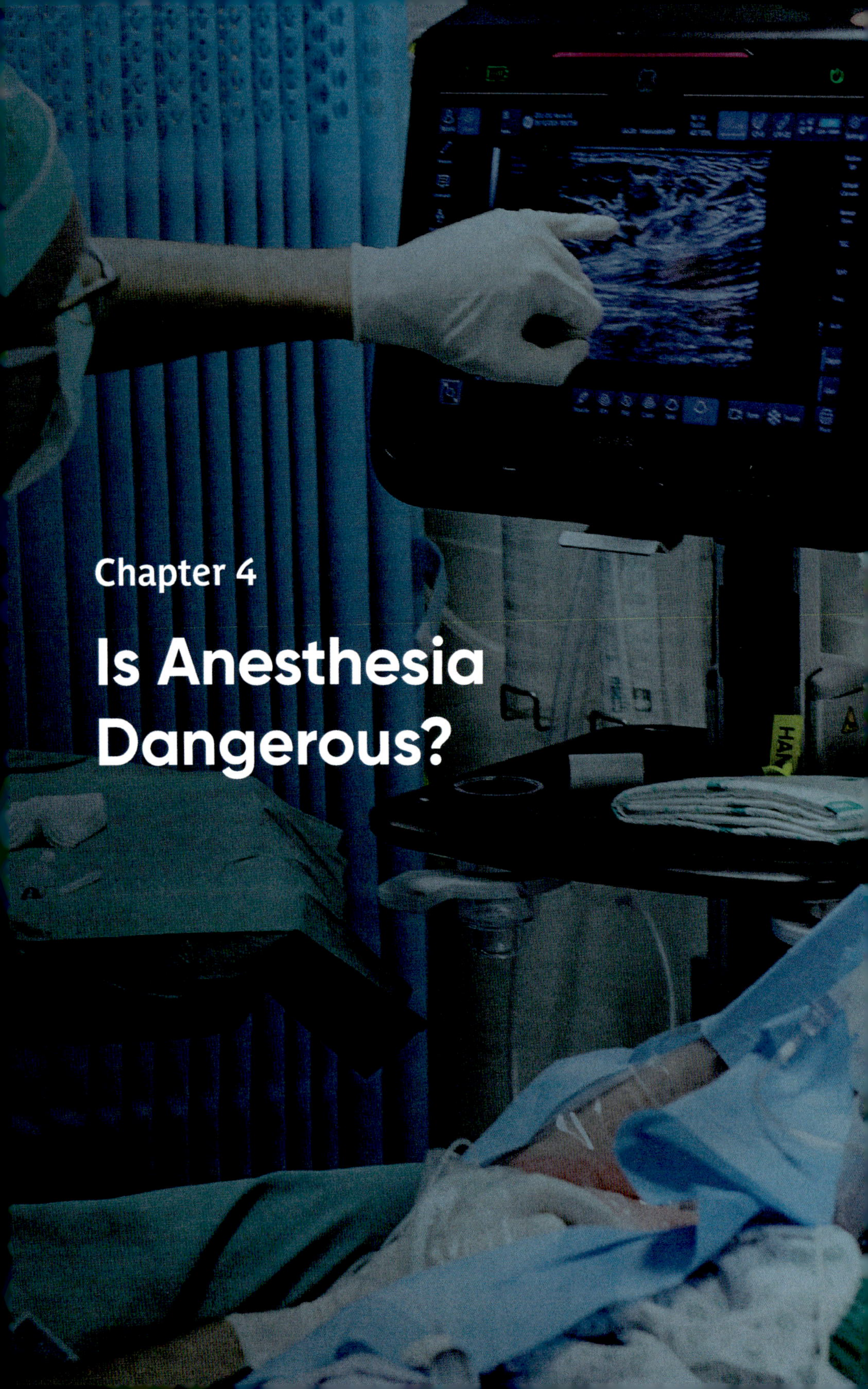

Chapter 4

Is Anesthesia Dangerous?

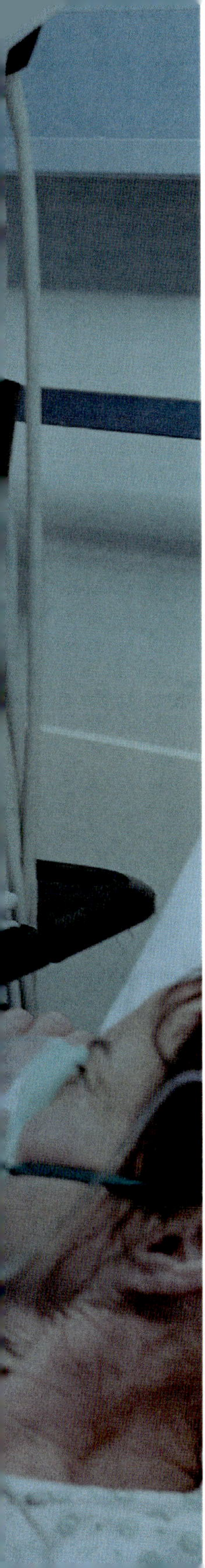

People ask this question more often than you might expect. Sometimes it's asked directly, with genuine concern. Sometimes it's disguised as a joke: "You'll put me to sleep and wake me up, right?", followed by a nervous laugh. And sometimes it's not asked at all, but you can see it in the patient's eyes as they sign the consent form.

So, is anesthesia dangerous? The honest answer is yes. And no.

I usually see the question arrive before it's spoken. The patient is sitting on the edge of the bed, wearing a gown that never quite closes in the back. The pen pauses for a moment above the signature line. They look up, not for reassurance, but for honesty.

That pause tells me everything. Anesthesia is one of the reasons modern medicine exists as we know it. Without it, surgery would be impossible. Pain, stress, and potential for physiologic collapse would make even routine procedures intolerable, and dangerous, as it was just a few decades ago. At the same time, anesthesia deliberately and profoundly interferes with the very systems that keep us alive: breathing, circulation, consciousness, reflexes.

We weaken them and make them highly vulnerable on highly elaborate purpose. That is where the risk lives. Every patient is different. Age, weight, genetics, comorbidities, medications, anxiety, previous experiences; each variable alters how the body responds. Two patients receiving the same anesthetic for the same procedure can behave in completely different ways. One sails through effortlessly. The other demands constant adjustment, vigilance, and intervention.

This variability is what makes anesthesia challenging-and why it can never be reduced to a formula. Anesthesiologists make complex decisions in real time. How deep anesthesia is deep enough? How much blood pressure can this patient tolerate? Is this change benign or the first sign of something serious? Which medication will stabilize without causing harm somewhere else?

Complications can and do occur. Blood pressure can drop suddenly. Hearts can misbehave. Airway can surprise you. A loose tooth. Allergic reactions appear without warning. Lungs stiffen. Oxygenation deteriorates. Sometimes, despite careful planning, things unravel faster than expected.

And then there is a fear patients rarely articulate but often carry: awareness during surgery. The idea of being conscious yet unable to move, of hearing voices or feeling pain during surgery. This is understandably frightening. Awareness under anesthesia can occur, but it is rare. Advances in monitoring, technique, and education have reduced its incidence dramatically. What has changed is both the risk itself, and the perception of it. Public awareness of this possibility has been amplified over the years, particularly after portrayals in popular culture such as the movie "Awake". While such depictions are dramatic and memorable, they do not reflect how modern anesthesia is practiced in reality.

Anesthesiologists carry this responsibility every day: not by dismissing fear, but by anticipating it, monitoring for it, and designing systems that make awareness increasingly rare. Still, "rare" is not "never," and that truth is never abstract to those who practice the specialty.

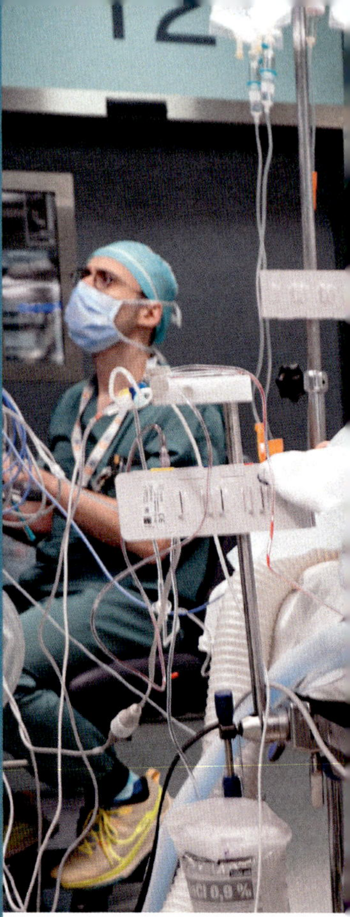

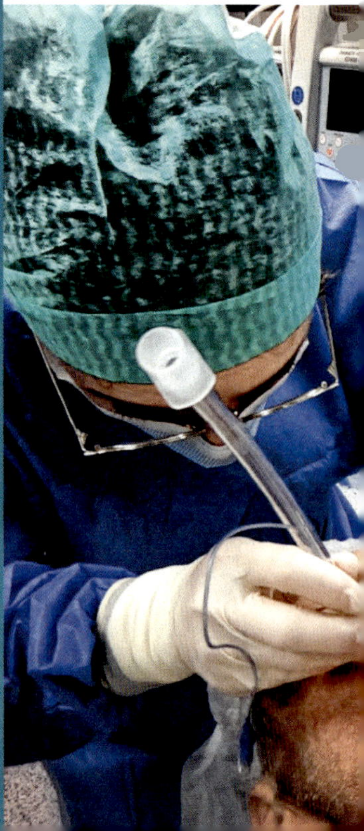

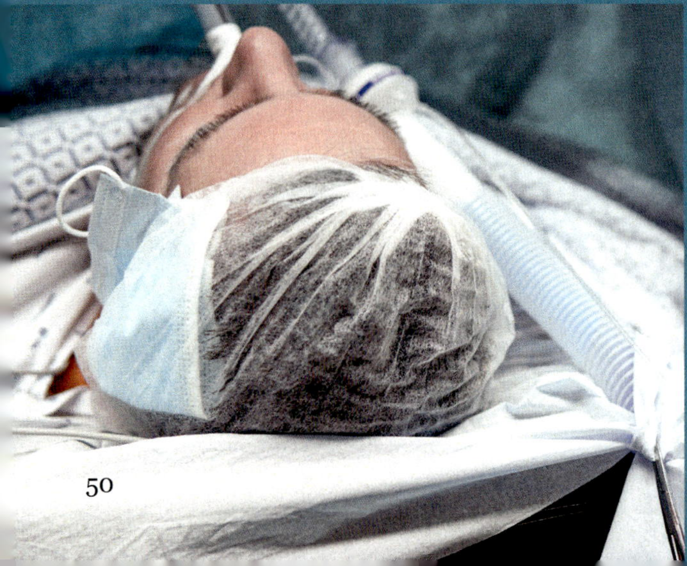

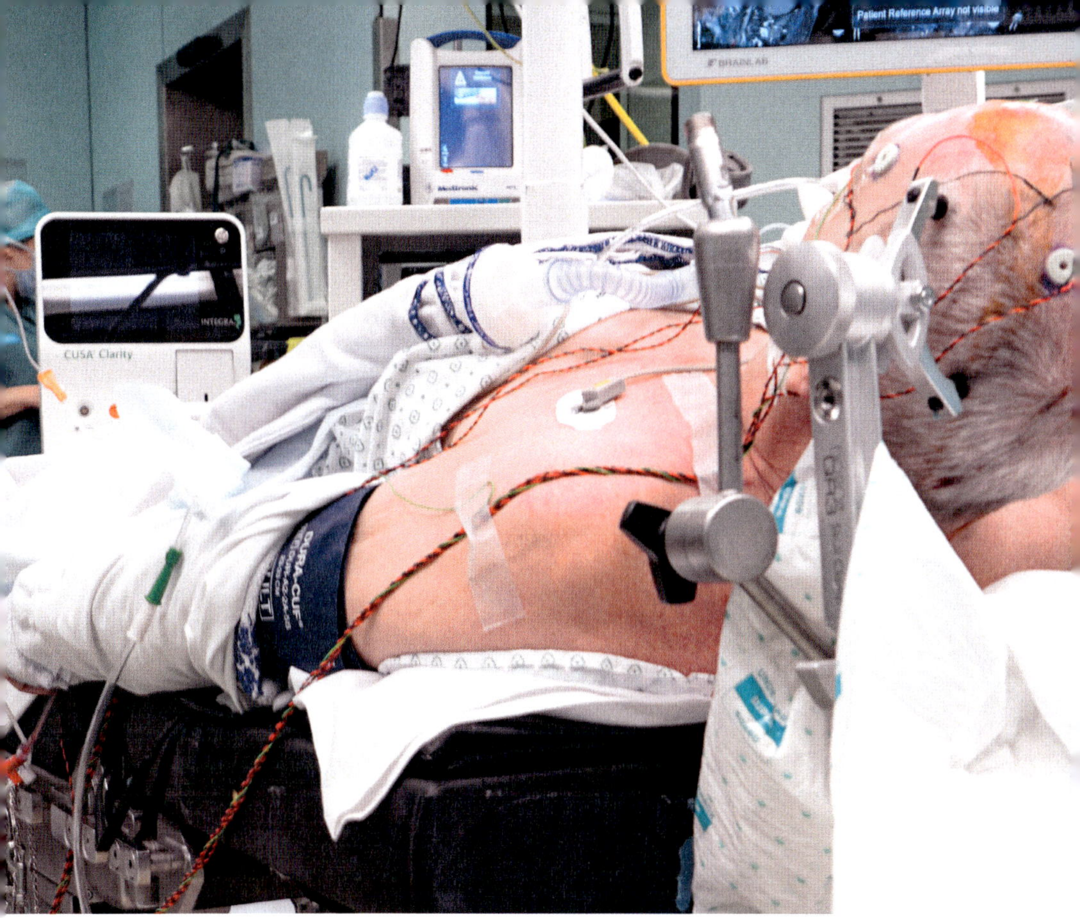
Patient Reference Array not visible
CUSA Clarity
INTEGRA
DURA-CUF

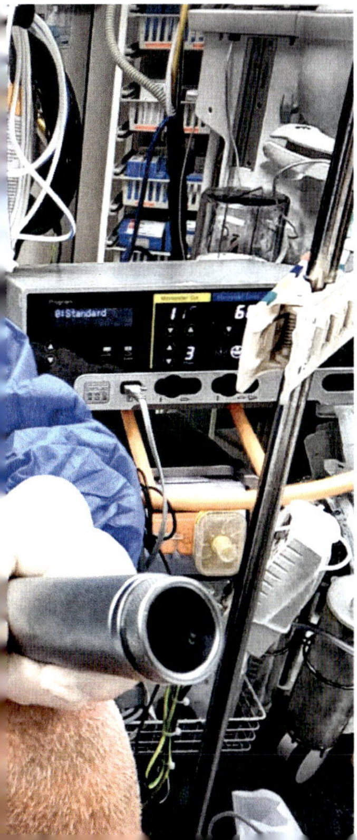
01Standard

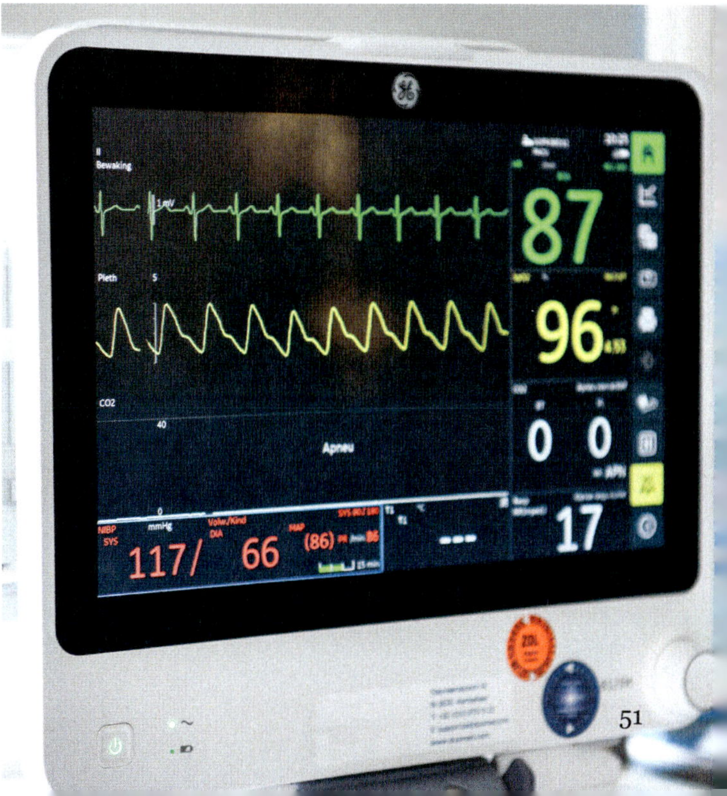
Bewaking
Pleth
CO2
Apneu
87
96
0
0
NIBP
mmHg
SYS
DIA
MAP
117/
66
(86)
17

I remember rushing emergency room gurneys soaked in blood from gunshot and knife wounds at St. Luke's - Roosevelt Hospital, in Spanish Harlem, New York where I worked for twenty or so years. Those moments forced decisions with no perfect answers. Administer too much anesthetic, and a patient who has already lost massive amounts of blood may not survive the anesthetic induction and mechanical ventilation, in which breathing is supported by a breathing machine. Administer too little, and the risk of awareness increases.

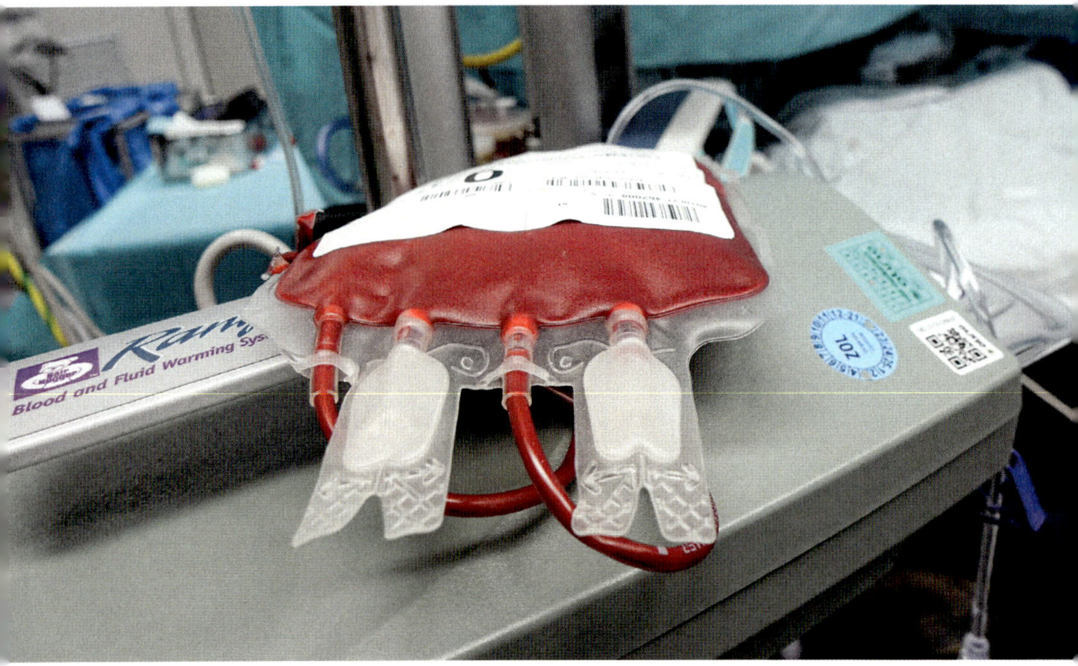

On more than one occasion, I leaned close and spoke quietly into patient's ear just before induction.

“I have a difficult decision to make,” I told them. ”I must balance keeping you alive with the risk that you may remember parts of what we are about to do. I will do what I believe gives you the best chance”. Even in the modern era of awareness monitoring, this consideration is still valid.

Then I proceeded with a deliberately reduced dose induction, combined with full neuromuscular blockade, enough to allow airway control and surgery without movement, while minimizing further physiologic collapse.

It is a choice no anesthesiologist makes lightly. Thankfully, none of those patients reported well documented recollection. But the memory of those moments remains, as a reminder of what the responsibility truly entails: choosing between imperfect options, under pressure, with another human life entirely dependent on your judgment.

That is the reality behind the reassurance patients hear. And it is why anesthesiologists take the fear of awareness seriously, not as a hypothetical, but as a responsibility that must be managed, case by case, moment by moment.

I have had patients ask me about awareness in a whisper, as if saying it aloud might make it more likely. I don't deflect the question. I explain what we do to prevent it, what we monitor, and what signs we watch for, because fear thrives in vagueness, and clarity is one of the safest drugs we have. So why does anesthesia work as well as it does?

Because anesthesiology is built around anticipating failure. We plan for complications that may never happen. We check equipment obsessively. We prepare backup plans for backup plans. We train for rare events until they feel familiar. We rehearse crises we hope never to encounter. This is not paranoia. It is professionalism.

Anesthesiology also relies on teamwork. Surgeons, nurses, technicians, and anesthesiologists function as a unit; communicating, adjusting, responding. When that coordination works well, risk is reduced dramatically. When it breaks down, even simple cases can become risky. That is where the calm of an anesthesiologist truly matters. In moments of uncertainty or crisis, the room often looks to the head of the bed for guidance. Calm is not a personality trait; it is a professional obligation.

I remember one of my early anesthesiology mentors, Dr Enio Gallozzi, advising me what to do when I was urgently called to the operating room.

Enio was Italian, trained in Europe, and arrived in New York in the early 1950s after a Fulbright fellowship in UK. He had seen enough medicine, and enough life to know that panic never helps. He grew up in Rome, and he carried that Roman street- level pragmatism with him: a calm exterior, sharp instincts, and a one-line answer for almost every situation. To us, he was a figure you went to for advice when things were complicated, less theatrical authority than quiet credibility, the kind of presence people trusted instinctively. Someone you listened to.

"Run like your life depends on it," he told me. "But when you reach the OR door, pause for a second. Take a breath. Then step in calmly."

Once inside, he taught, the first task is not action but organization. Ask a simple question: "What's the problem?", and ask it calmly. That alone quiets the room. From there, restore order: assign roles, prioritize tasks, and bring everyone's attention back to the one thing that matters most, helping the patient.

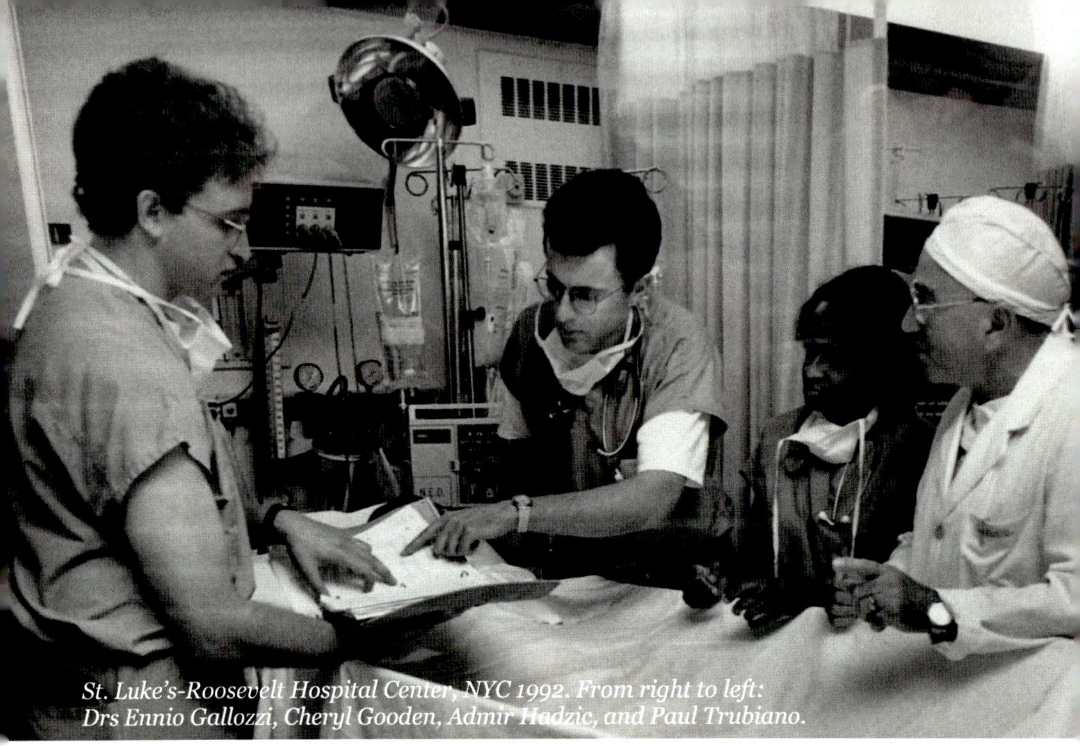

St. Luke's-Roosevelt Hospital Center, NYC 1992. From right to left: Drs Ennio Gallozzi, Cheryl Gooden, Admir Hadzic, and Paul Trubiano.

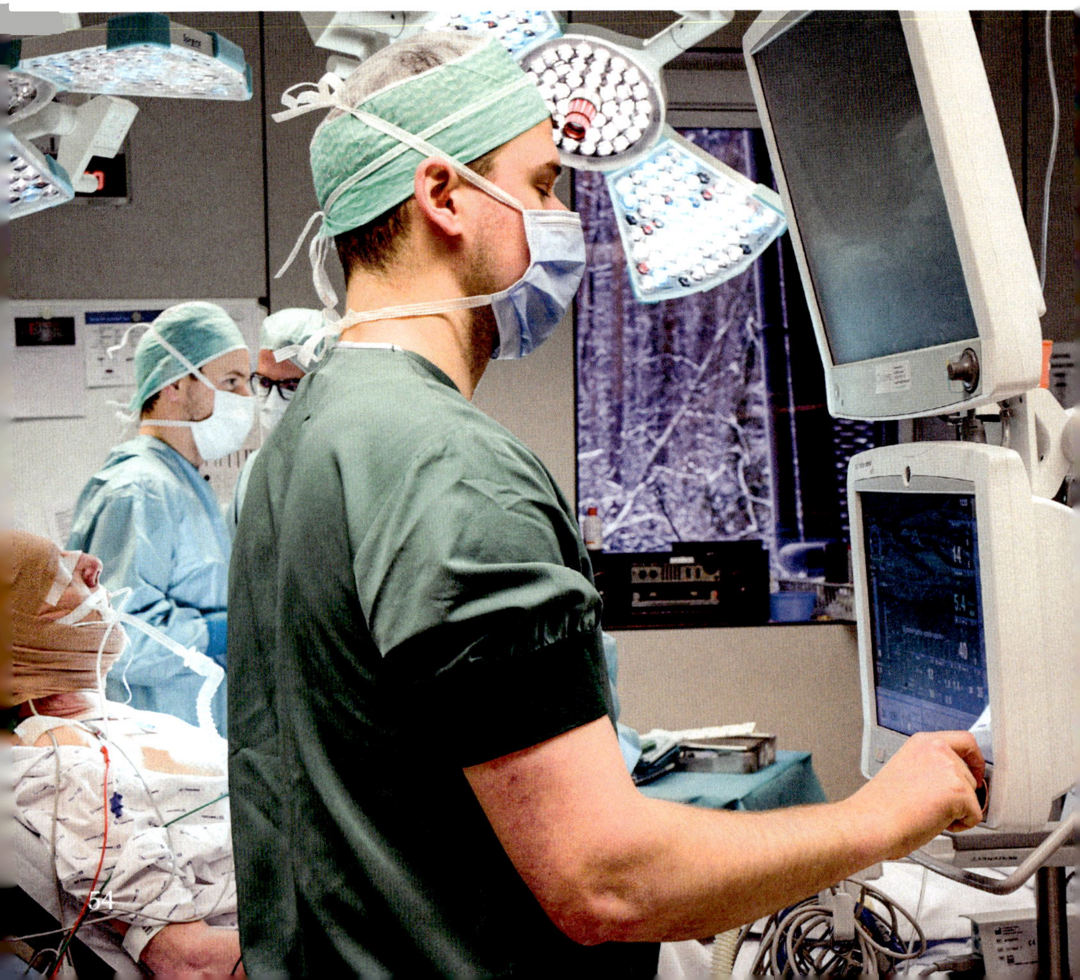

That lesson stayed with me. In anesthesia, your composure sets the tone. When you slow down, the room follows. When disarray settles, teamwork resets to a coordinated effort directed toward a single goal. And that is often what turns a complication into a recovery.

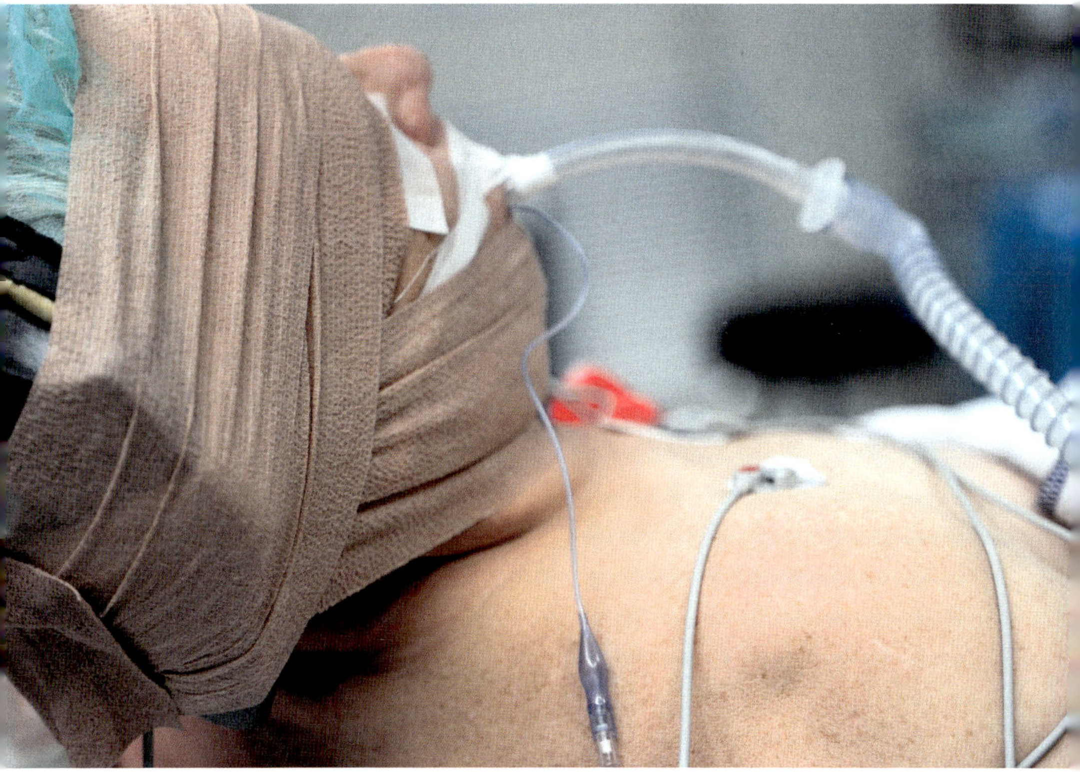

Over the years, safety in anesthesia has improved enormously. Monitoring is better. Medications are more precise. Education is more standardized.

Outcomes are vastly improved compared to decades ago. Yet the fundamental truth remains: anesthesia will never be risk-free.

When a patient hands over consciousness, they place themselves in a position of absolute vulnerability. They trust that someone will notice the subtle change before it becomes catastrophic. That someone will act quickly, correctly, and calmly when things don't go according to plan. Anesthesiology is dangerous in the same way flying is dangerous, because it involves complex systems operating close to their limits. The safety does not come from the absence of risk. It comes from respect for it.

So, when patients ask me whether anesthesia is dangerous, I tell them this: it is safe not because nothing can go wrong, but because someone is always watching for the moment it might.

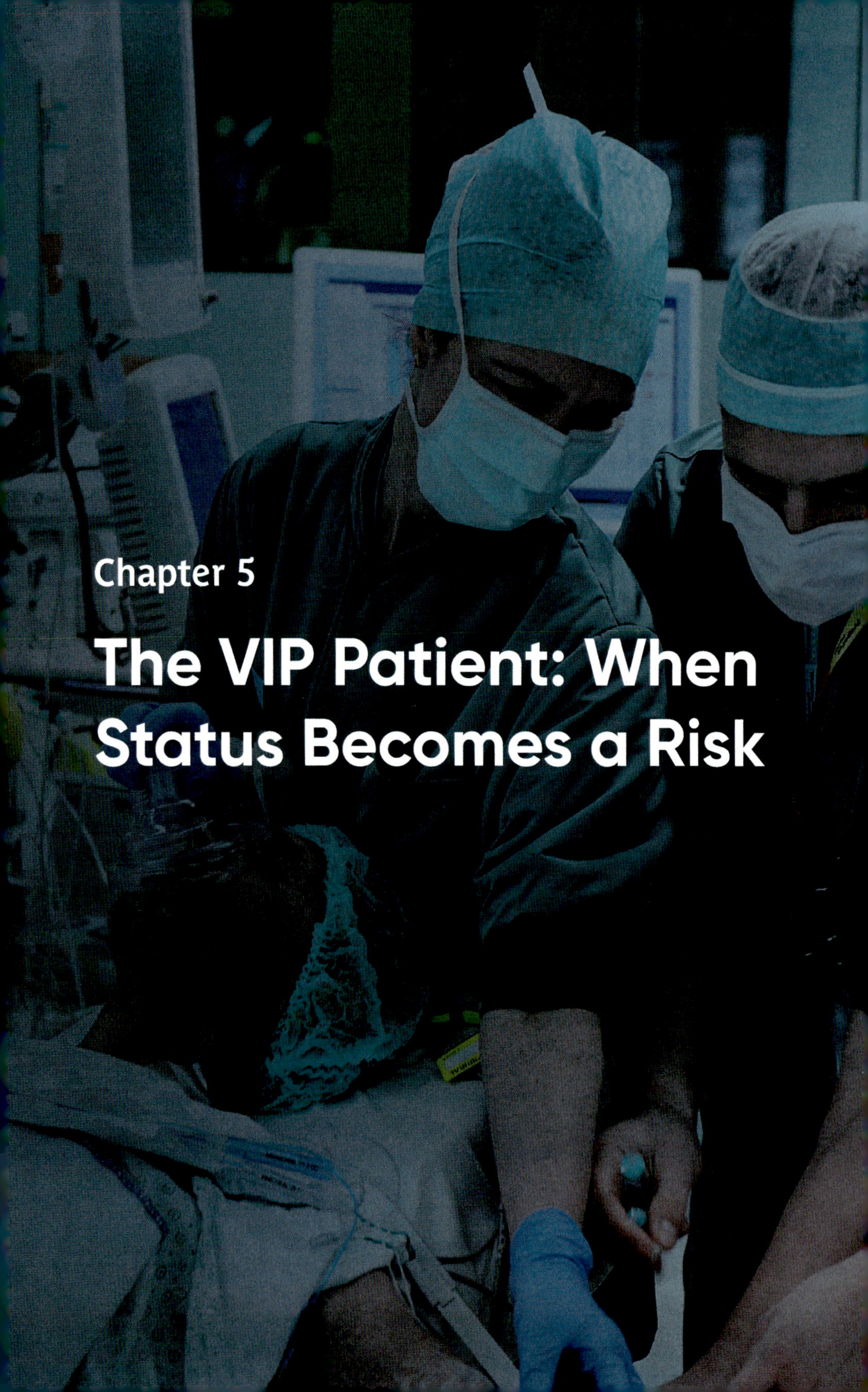

Chapter 5

The VIP Patient: When Status Becomes a Risk

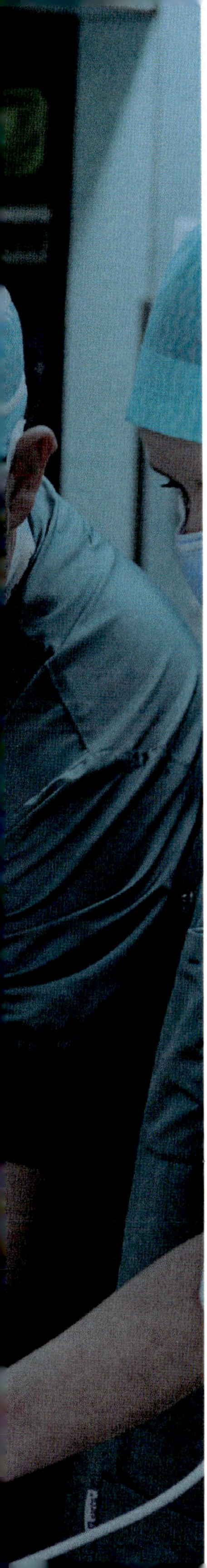

“Do you know who I am?”

Every anesthesiologist hears some version of this question eventually. Sometimes it comes directly from the patient spoken with confidence. Sometimes it arrives indirectly, through a secretary, a hospital administrator, a colleague, or a subtle hint about status, influence, or expectations. The implication is always the same: this patient is different, “special”.

In the practice of anesthesiology, VIP patients are not rare. They are politicians, celebrities, executives, donors, colleagues, or family members of people who matter. They are often anxious, not unreasonably so because anesthesia requires surrendering control. And when people who are used to control lose it, fear surfaces quickly.

Ironically, that fear is where danger begins. There is a powerful temptation to treat VIP patients differently. To offer something “extra.” To choose what sounds like the best, newest, most impressive technique. To skip routine steps that feel inconvenient when treating a VIP. To add tests that reassure everyone involved even if they add little value.

It feels respectful. It often isn’t.

One of the quiet lessons of anesthesiology is this: special treatment is not always better treatment. In fact, it can be worse.

The best anesthesia is not the most exotic one. It is the one you perform well, consistently, and often. A technically elegant regional block done by an occasional practitioner of local anesthesia is riskier than a straightforward general anesthetic delivered by someone who does just that. Expertise in anesthesiology is not theoretical, it is earned through repetition.

VIP syndrome occurs when objectivity slips.

When treating a VIP, doctors sometimes tend to hesitate to follow standard protocols. They second-guess themselves. They invite too many voices. They avoid saying "no." The usual clarity of decision-making becomes clouded by fear of scrutiny, reputation, or consequence.

With VIP patients, the atmosphere changes. Titles and advisors fill the room. Questions accelerate, suggestions increase, and while reassurance is demanded, responsibility becomes diffuse.

That is the moment anesthesiology demands discipline.

History offers painful examples of what happens when VIP syndrome takes hold. Fame, wealth, and access do not guarantee good medical care. Sometimes they guarantee the opposite: too many opinions, too little accountability, no single person clearly in charge.

Anesthesiology does not tolerate that ambiguity.At the head of the bed, someone must decide. Someone must commit. Someone must take responsibility - not just for the plan, but for its execution. That responsibility becomes even heavier when the patient is a colleague.

Doctors make difficult patients. They know just enough to be afraid. They request specific medications, specific techniques. Even though they may not use the same medications and techniques in their own daily clinical care for others.

One of the most important skills an anesthesiologist develops is the ability to say, calmly and without apology: this is how we do it safely here.

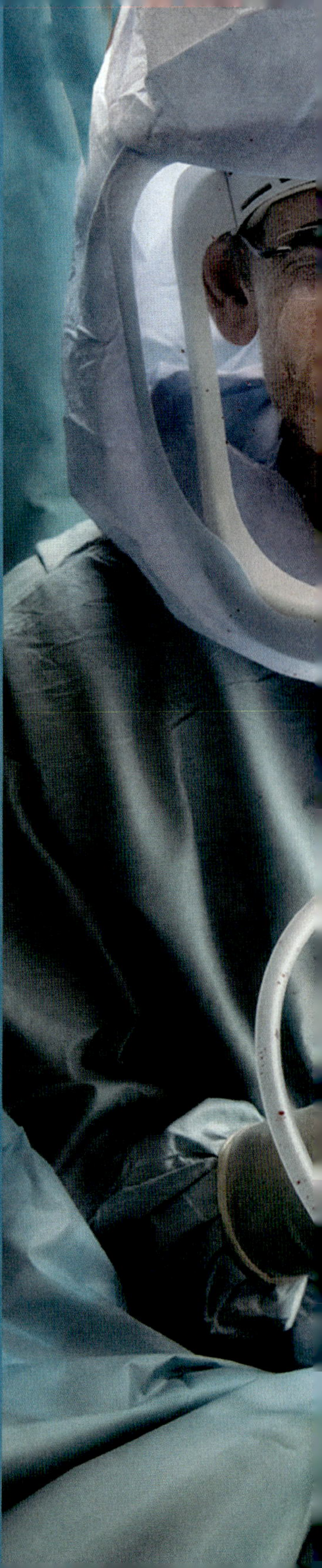

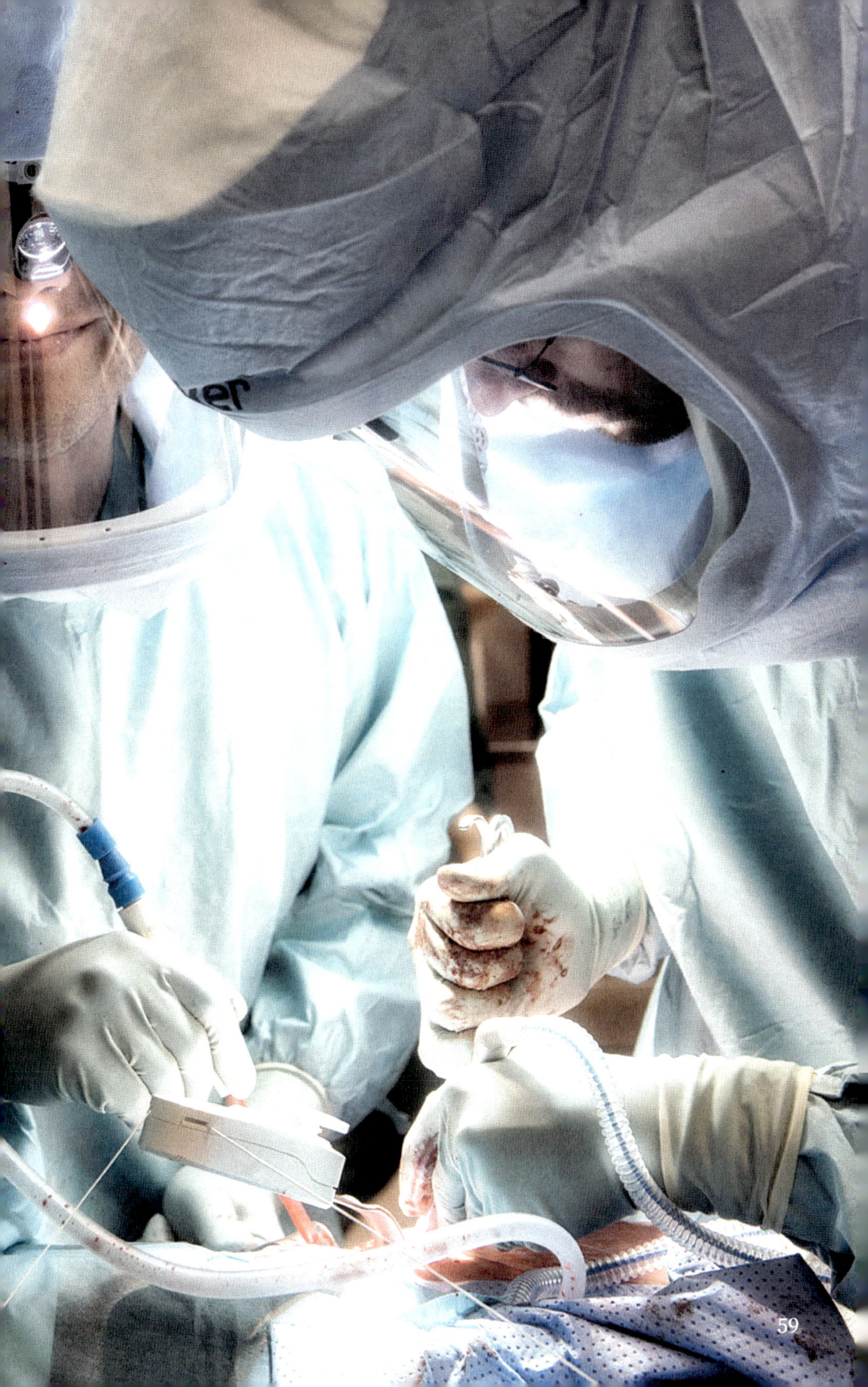

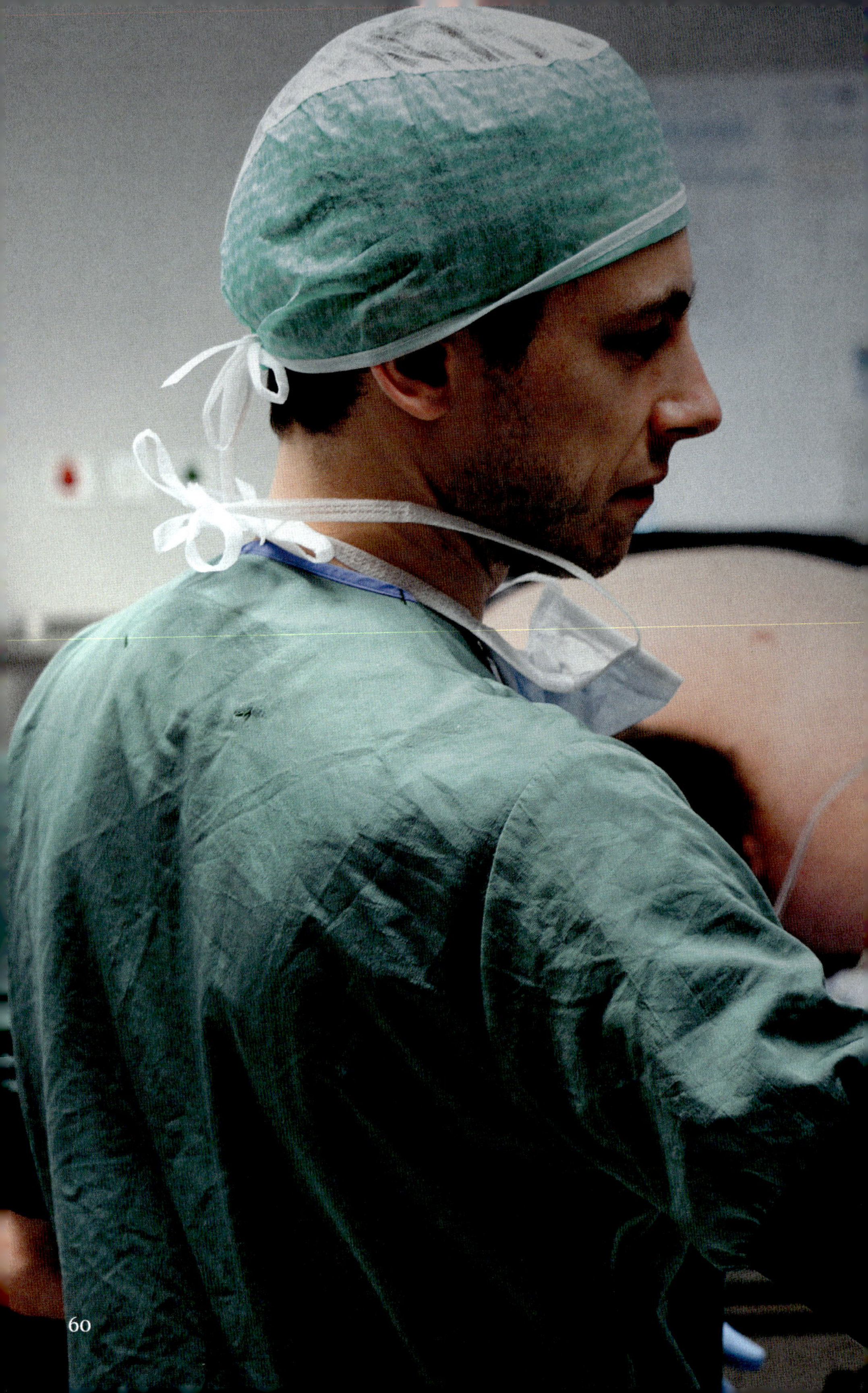

The same checks. The same preparation. The same standards.

VIP patients deserve excellent care. But excellent care is not personalized indulgence. It is disciplined consistency. When anesthesia goes well, no one remembers the technique. They remember that they woke up safely. That they were comfortable. That nothing went wrong. That outcome has nothing to do with fame.

When I needed shoulder surgery, my fellows and staff asked me the two questions anesthesiologists always ask colleagues who become patients: What kind of anesthesia do you want? And who do you want to do it? I answered by asking them a question in return: What do we routinely do for patients undergoing this operation? They answered without hesitation, "an interscalene brachial plexus catheter". And who performs it for our patients? I asked. "We do," they said. "The fellows." That settled it.

That was exactly what I wanted for my surgery: an interscalene catheter, performed by the same trainees who did it every day for our patients. Because it was practiced, standardized, and done well in our hospital. If you believe in your system, you trust it, especially when you or the VIP are the one on the table.

The operating room is a great equalizer. Under anesthesia, every patient breathes the same oxygen. Every heart responds to the same physiology. Every mistake carries the same consequences.

Anesthesiology does not care who you are.

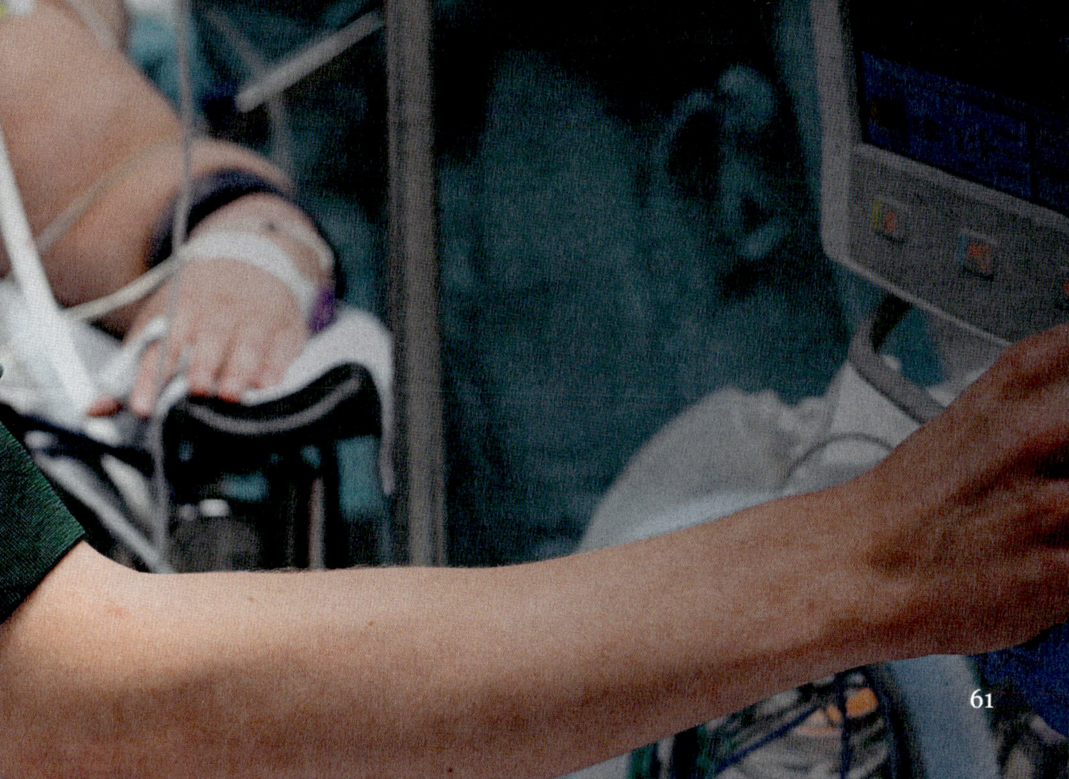

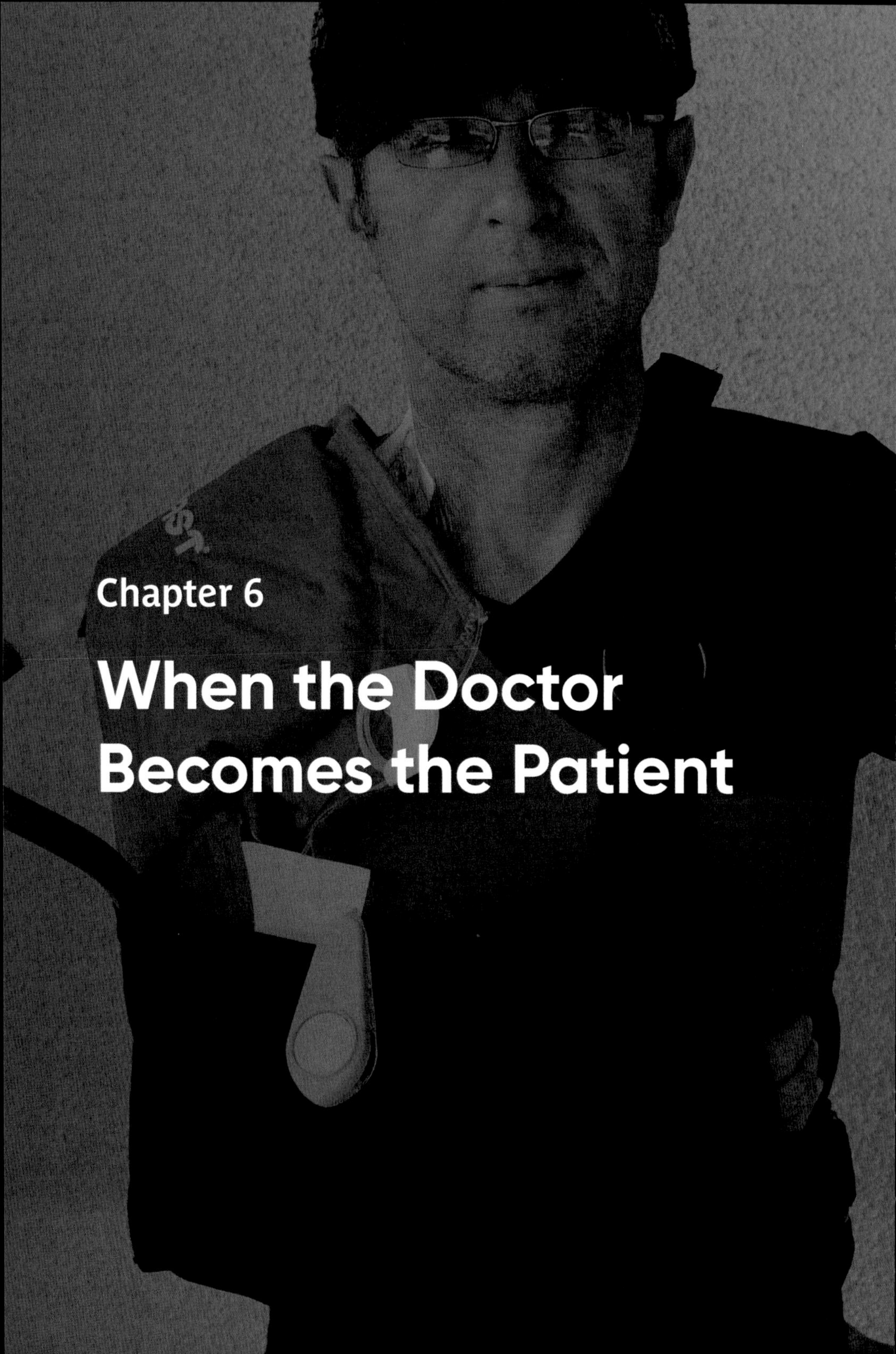

Chapter 6

When the Doctor Becomes the Patient

Every anesthesiologist has opinions about anesthesia. Often very strong ones. We debate techniques, medications, monitors, and protocols endlessly. We argue about evidence, experience, and nuance. We teach what we believe works best. We critique what doesn't. And quietly, each of us carries a private answer to an unspoken question:

What anesthesia would I choose for myself?

A few years ago, I had the opportunity to find out. During a fencing (epee, a sport I trained in NYC) competition, I felt something snap in my shoulder. After the snap my weapon - holding right arm became useless. Days later, an MRI confirmed what I fearfully suspected: a rotator cuff tear. Surgery was inevitable.

On the morning of the operation, I arrived at St. Luke's-Roosevelt Hospital in New York, not as the anesthesiologist, but as the patient. That role reversal can be disorienting and intimidating. You notice small things you usually ignore. The way the operating room feels too bright and too cold at the same time. The cold feel of adhesive of ECG stickers and the feeling of tugging when you shift your shoulder. The monitor tone that you normally treat as background suddenly sounding personal.

I was received by my colleague Dr. Jeff Gadsden who supervised Drs Kim Gratestein and Colleen McCally. My trainees, fellows. People I had taught, supervised, and trusted with patients for years. After the initial greetings, they asked me the two questions anesthesiologists always ask colleagues who become patients:

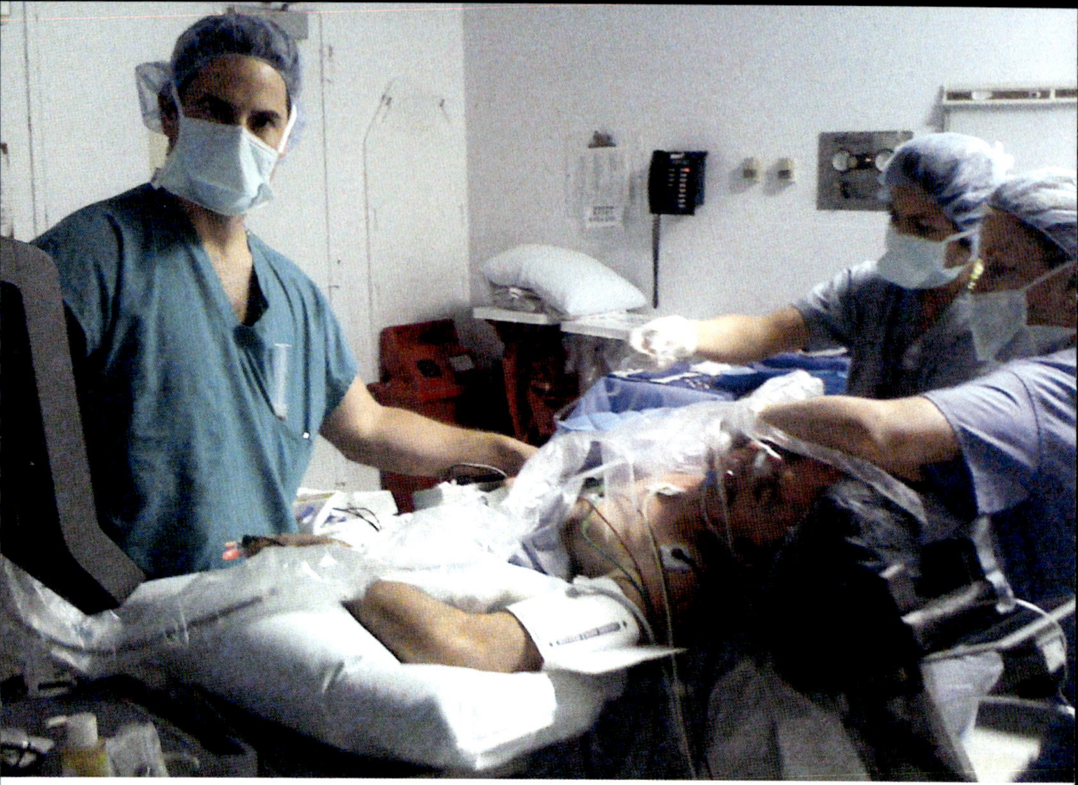

“What kind of anesthesia do you want?” “And who should do it?” My answer surprised no one. “Whatever we give to patients here, that’s what I’ll have.”

At that institution, every patient undergoing shoulder surgery received an interscalene brachial plexus block. Many received a continuous catheter, providing analgesia for days after surgery. It was standardized, practiced daily, and executed well.

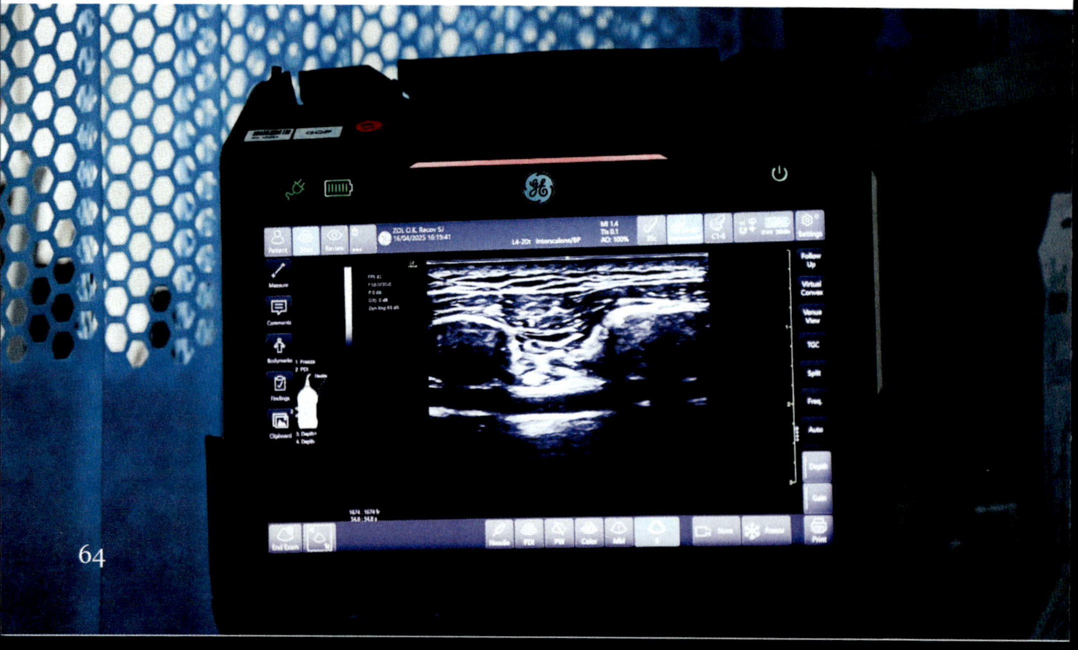

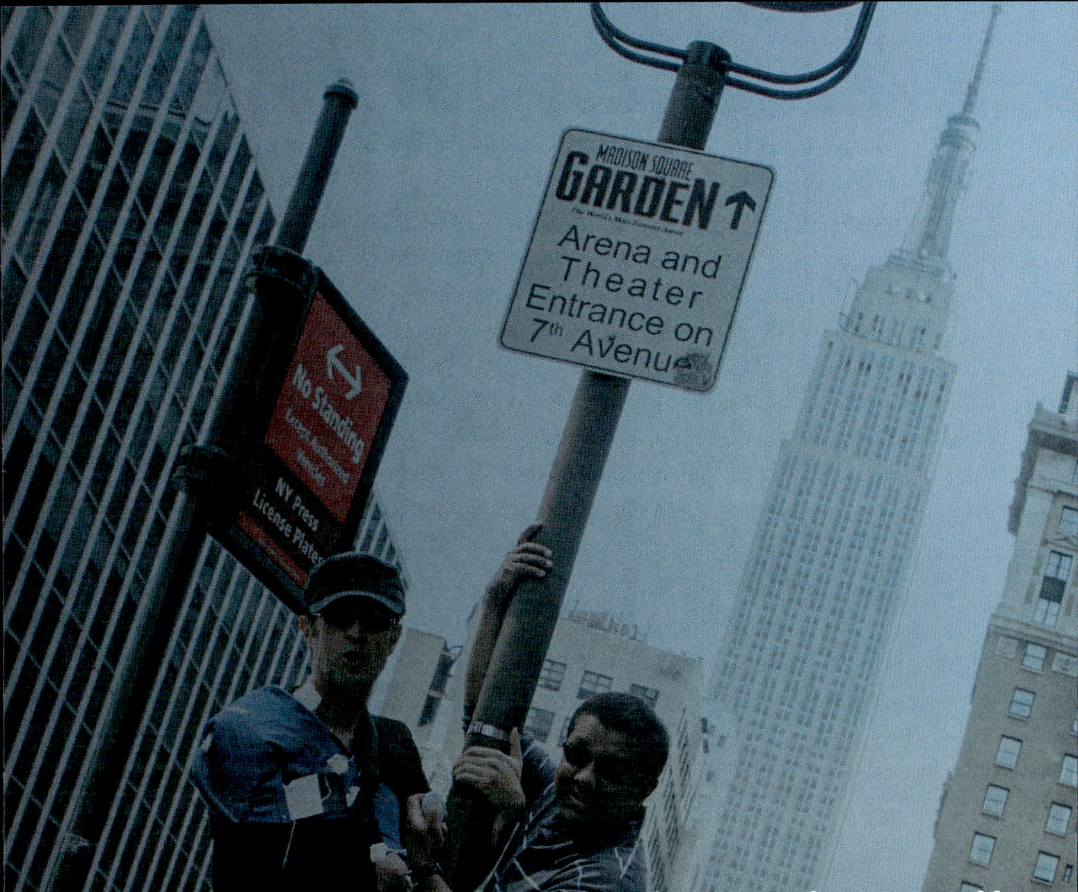

If you train people properly, you should trust them. This was not bravado. It was a statement of belief in education, repetition, and systems that work.

The anesthetic block was performed smoothly under ultrasound guidance. I was awake, calm, and fully aware of what was happening, watching hands move with confidence, recognizing the choreography I had seen thousands of times from the other side. There is a peculiar moment when you feel the last normal sensation fade and realize, that you are no longer in control, and you are choosing to be okay with that.

When the surgery began, I could see the operative field on the screen while feeling absolutely no pain. It was surreal.

I arrived at the hospital at 8 a.m. By 10 a.m., my rotator cuff had been repaired, and I was sitting in a car, being driven to a shopping mall to buy clothes, because when else does a busy clinician have time to shop, if not when his dominant arm is temporarily out of service?

That evening, we hosted friends from overseas. The next day, catheter still in place and arm immobilized, I joined them sightseeing around New York. Pain was not part of the story.

If I had to do it again, would I choose the same anesthetic technique? Without hesitation.

Experiences like this are difficult to capture in formal studies. Clinical trials measure outcomes like mortality, length of stay, or complications at 30 or 60 days. They struggle to quantify what patients actually feel: comfort, confidence, autonomy, the ability to resume life quickly and without fear.

But as patients, we remember those things vividly. Becoming the patient reinforced something I had believed for years: good anesthesia is not just about survival. It is about quality of experience. About enabling recovery, not merely enduring it. And perhaps most Importantly, that experi-

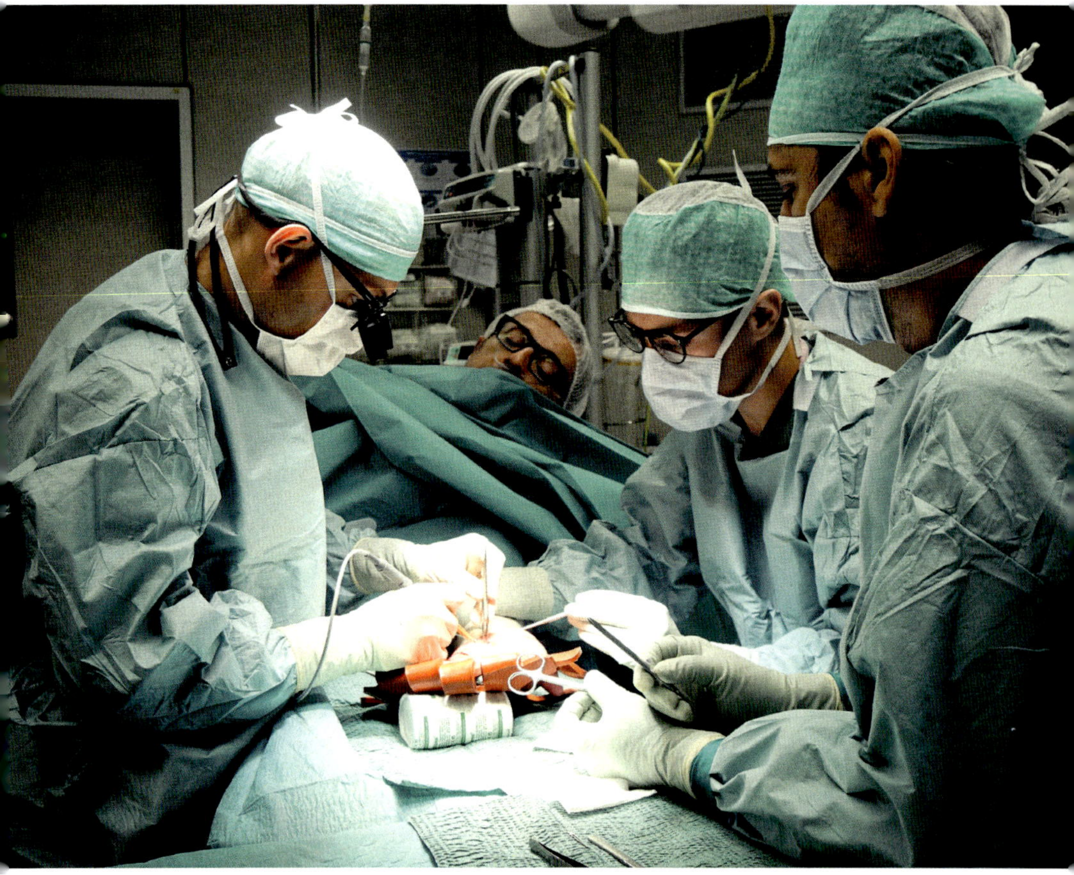

ence, being a patient, reaffirmed the power of trust.

Trust in systems. Do not choose a different, "special" anesthetic treatment for your own operation than what you do every day for patients.

Trust in techniques practiced daily, not occasionally. Because when it's your own body on the table, theory fades quickly.

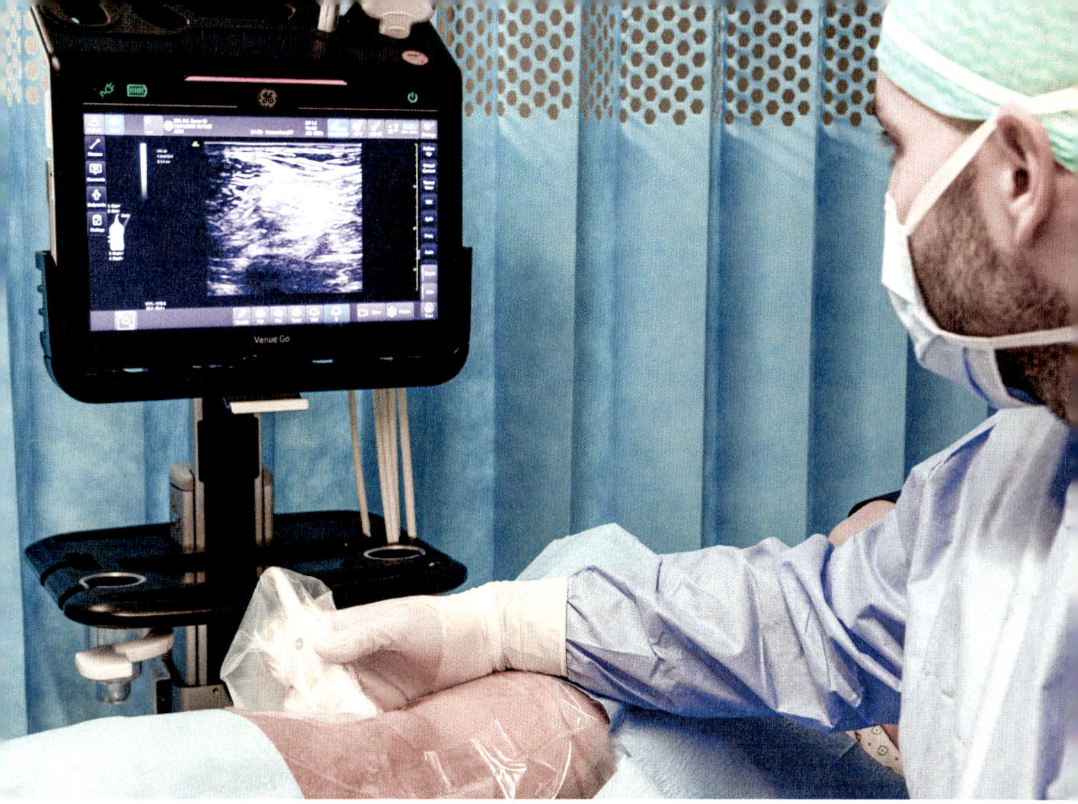
Venue Go

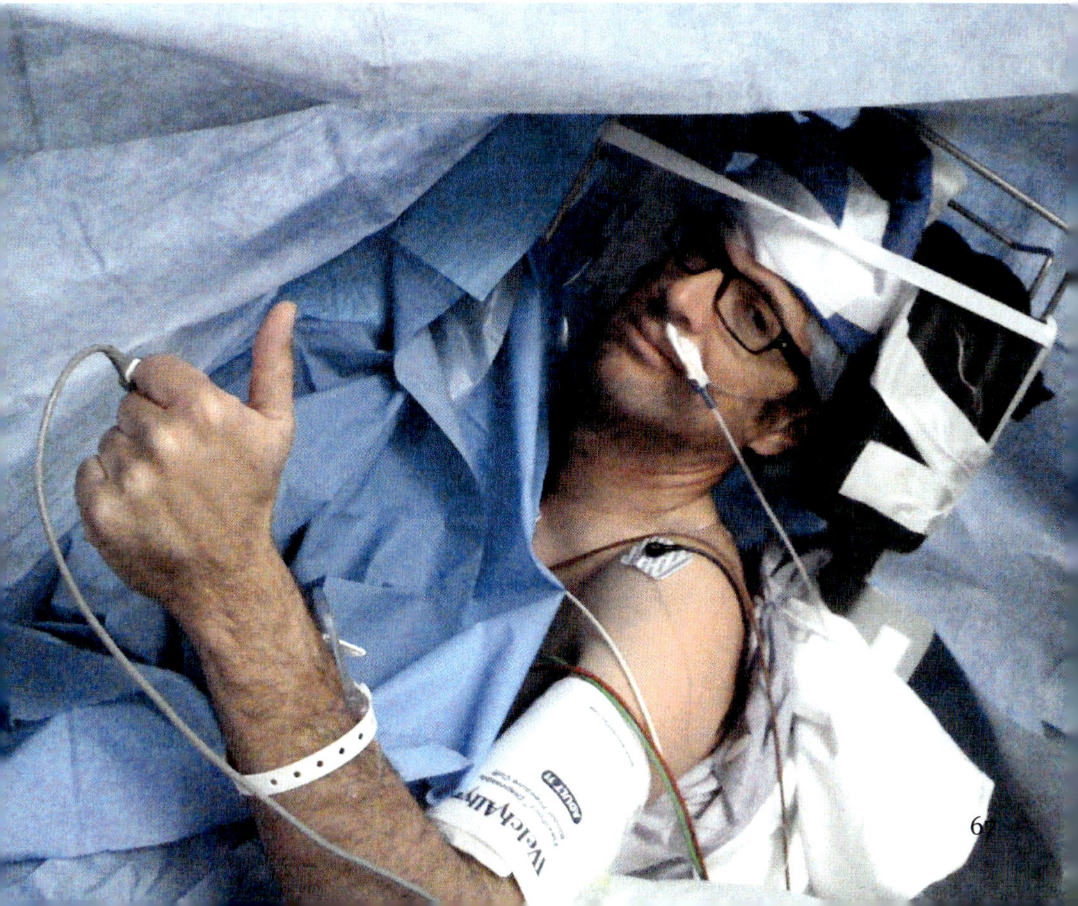
Welch Allyn

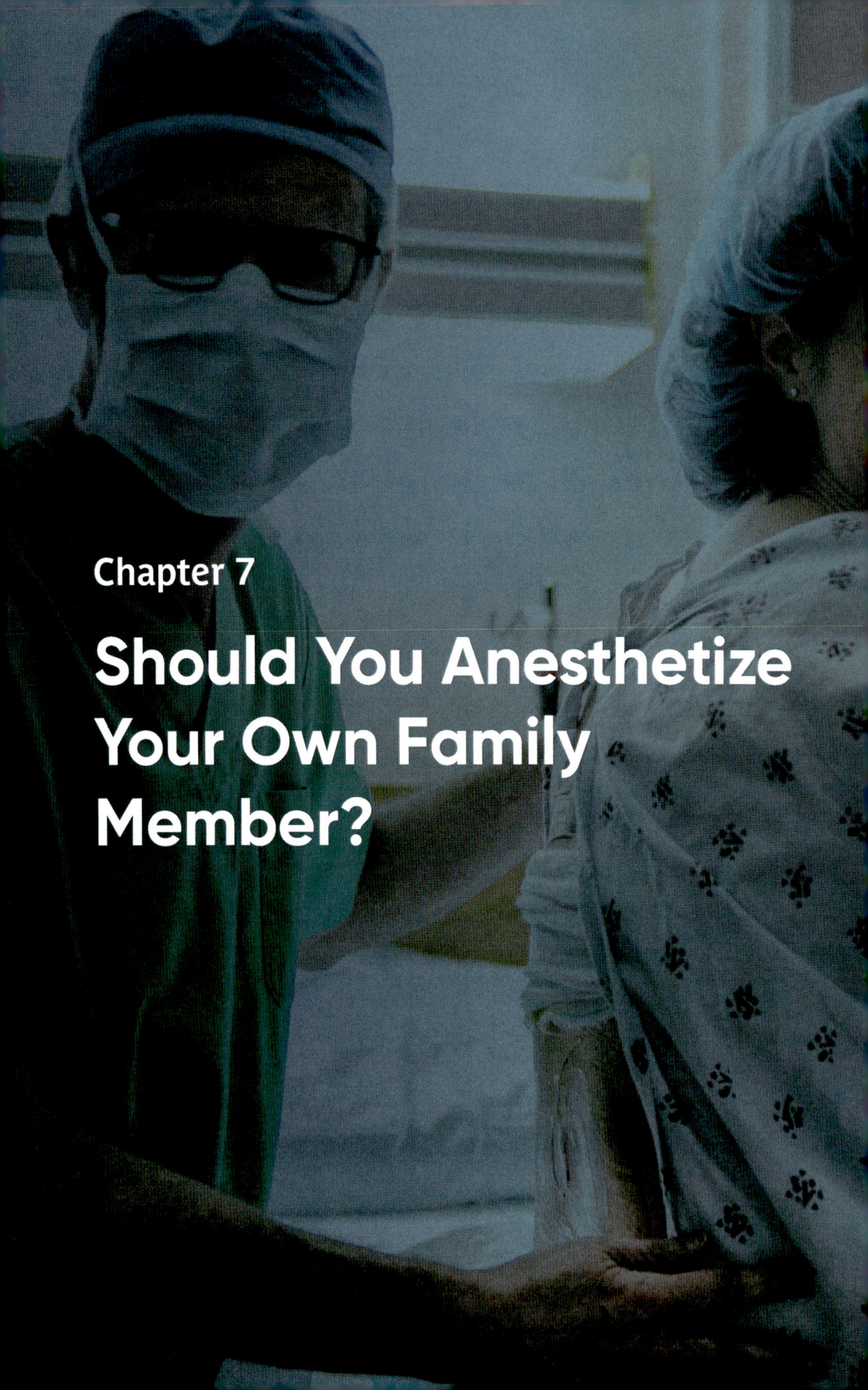

Chapter 7

Should You Anesthetize Your Own Family Member?

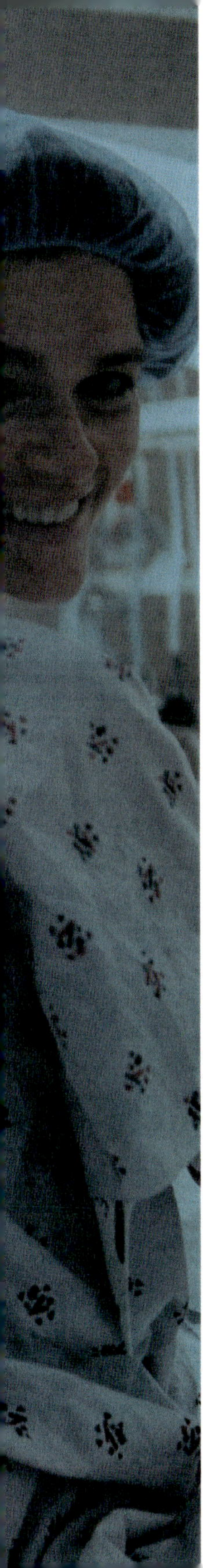

Every anesthesiologist is asked this question at some point. Sometimes by friends. Sometimes by colleagues. And sometimes, far more quietly, by themselves. So, should you be the anesthesiologist for your own family?

On the surface, it sounds logical. Who would care more? Who would be more vigilant? Who would know the risks, the nuances, the shortcuts, and the traps; better than you? And yet, medicine has long warned us against treating those closest to us. Not because we lack skill, but because we lack something just as important: distance. Objectivity is one of anesthesia's most powerful tools. It allows you to make clean decisions under pressure. To say no when needed. To follow protocol when emotion tempts deviation. To choose what is right, not what feels comforting in the moment.

Family changes that equation.

When the patient is someone you love, every monitor alarm feels louder. Every blood pressure fluctuation feels personal. The internal dialogue becomes more complex: Is this normal? Am I overreacting? Am I missing something?

There is also the weight of consequence. If something goes wrong, how do you carry that forward into family life? How do you separate professional judgment from personal responsibility when the two collide?

For these reasons, many anesthesiologists choose not to anesthetize their own family members. And many doctors opt out of treating their family as patients. They prefer to stand back, to trust a colleague, to remain present as a partner, a child, a parent rather than as the one at the head of the bed.

And yet. Life, as it often does, presents moments that don't fit neatly into guidelines. A few years back, 2014, at Roosevelt Hospital in New York City, my wife Catherine, was delivering our first child, Adriana.I remember that evening with absolute clarity. We were at a casual dinner with friends on Manhattan's East Side when Catherine caught my eye across the table and, almost imperceptibly, mouthed, "I think my water broke". It felt unreal, too soon, nearly a month early. We excused ourselves, hearts racing, and drove through the city to Roosevelt Hospital on Amsterdam and 57th, a place I knew professionally but had never entered like this. After examining her, our obstetrician, Dr. Ed Jew, paused, smiled gently, and said, "We're going to have a baby tonight."

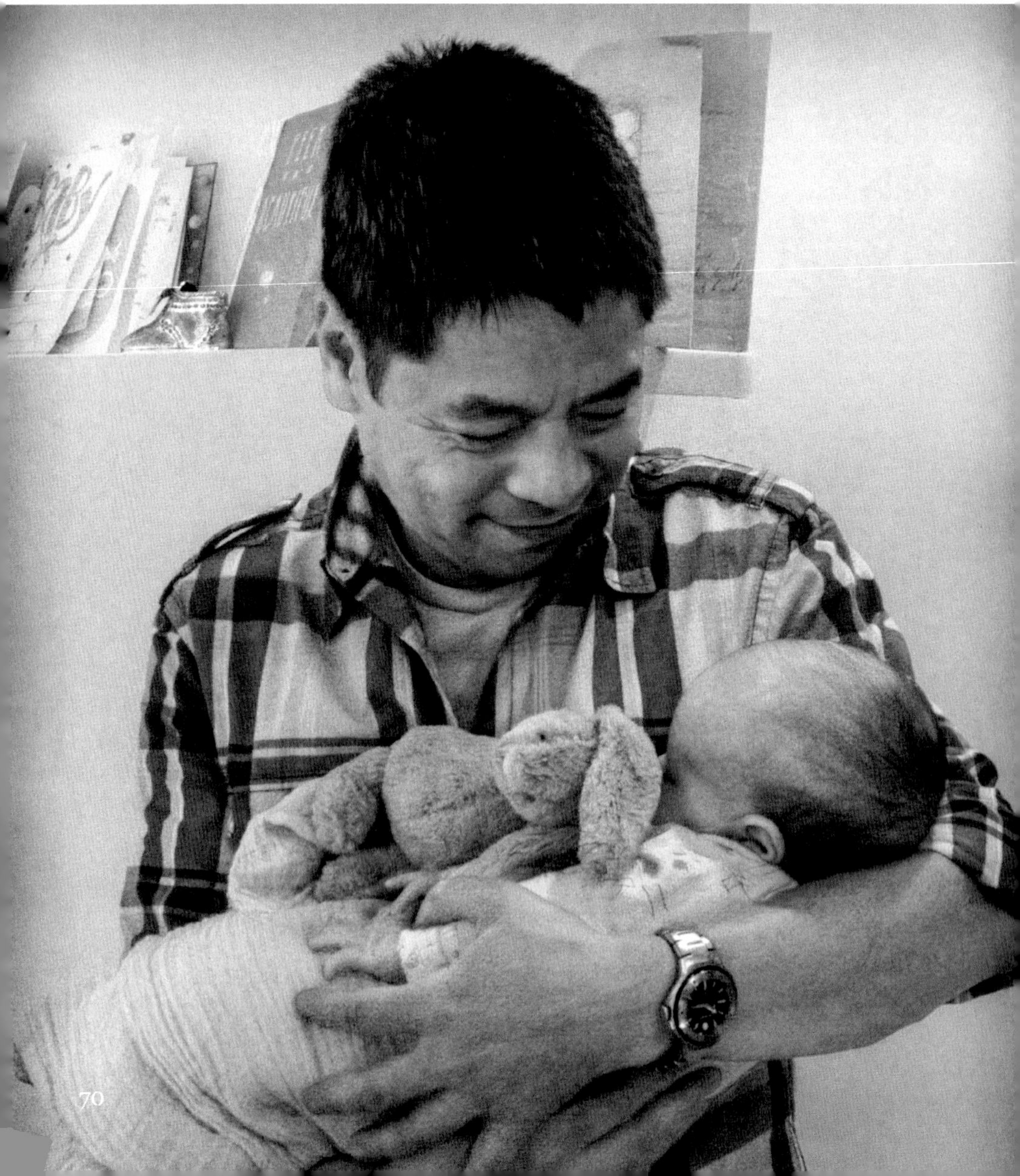

We were anxious in the way only parents always are, especially with the first time baby. The hospital was familiar to me. The staff were colleagues. The environment felt safe. And the question arose; not formally, not ceremonially, but naturally: Would I give her the epidural? In that moment, theory gave way to trust.

I knew the setting. I knew the team. I knew the plan. Most importantly, I knew my limits. I wasn't there to

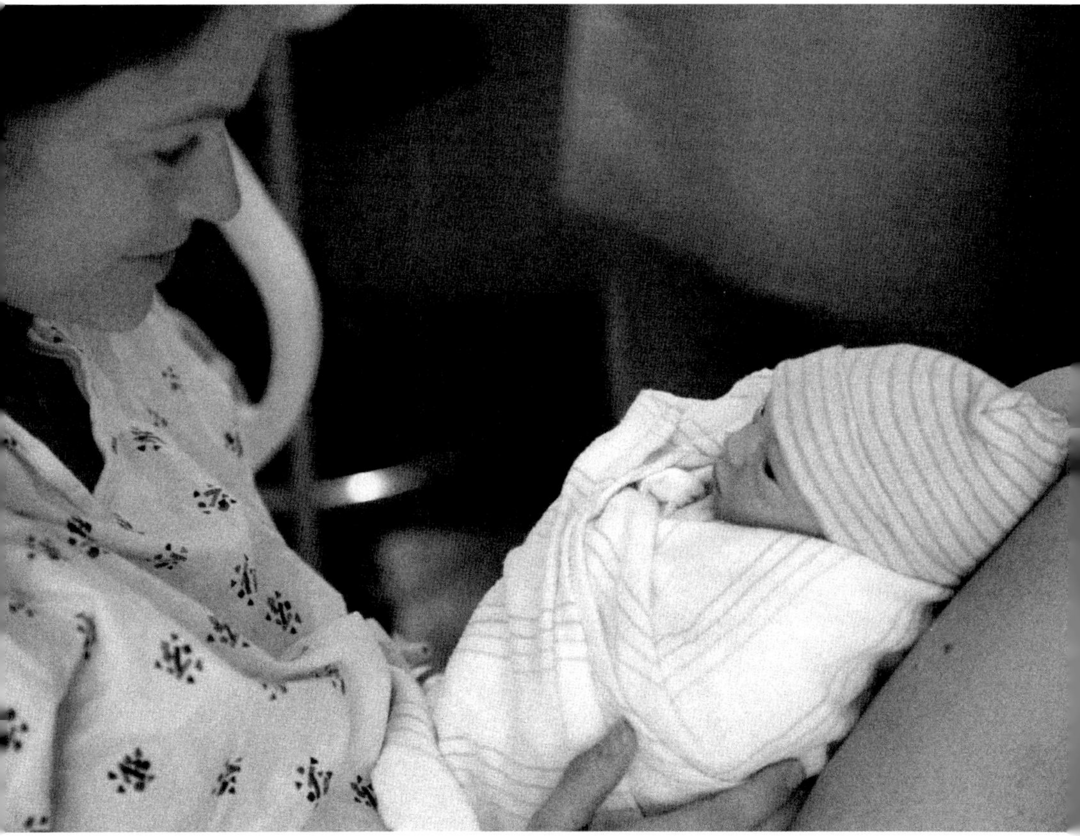

be heroic or exceptional. I was there to be precise, calm, and restrained; to do exactly what I had done many times before.

So yes, I gave anesthesia to my wife for the birth of our daughter. It was one of the most emotionally complex moments of my professional life. At the head of the bed stood not just an anesthesiologist, but a husband. A future father. A man acutely aware that the two people he loved most depended on his skill and composure.

I remember a brief second that felt anything but ordinary: the way my glove gripped the epidural syringe as advanced it toward the epidural space. The monitor's steady beeping continuing as if nothing special was happening, and Catherine slouched in position for the procedure with that particular combination of trust and fear that no textbook prepares you for.

And yet, something remarkable happens when training is deep enough. The hands know what to do. Muscle memory takes over. The same checks. The same vigilance. The same respect for anatomy and physiology. Emotion does not disappear, but it quiets, making room for focus. For care. For presence.

When Adriana was born, healthy and crying, something shifted permanently in me. I had seen thousands of births before. But this one rewired my understanding of trust.

I understood, viscerally, what we ask of patients and families every day. To surrender control. To believe that the person behind the mask will notice everything that matters. To trust that love and professionalism can coexist, when handled with humility. But would I recommend that every anesthesiologist anesthetize their own family? The Answer: No!

There is no universal answer. But I do believe this: whether you are at the head of the bed or standing beside it, being an anesthesiologist changes how you experience those moments forever. You see the fragility more clearly. You respect the stakes more deeply. And you never forget that behind every monitor is a family trusting someone they may never truly know.

Sometimes, that someone is you.

And sometimes, the most professional choice is knowing when it shouldn't be.

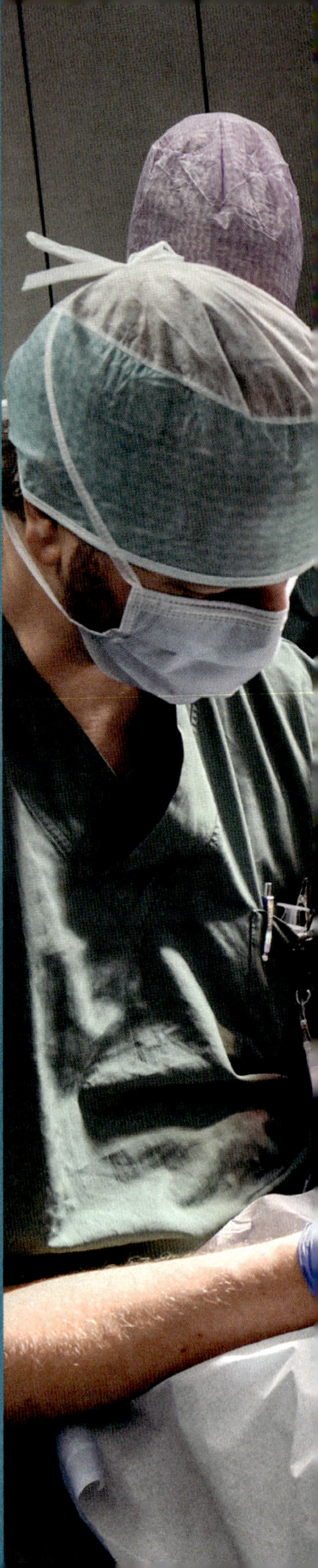

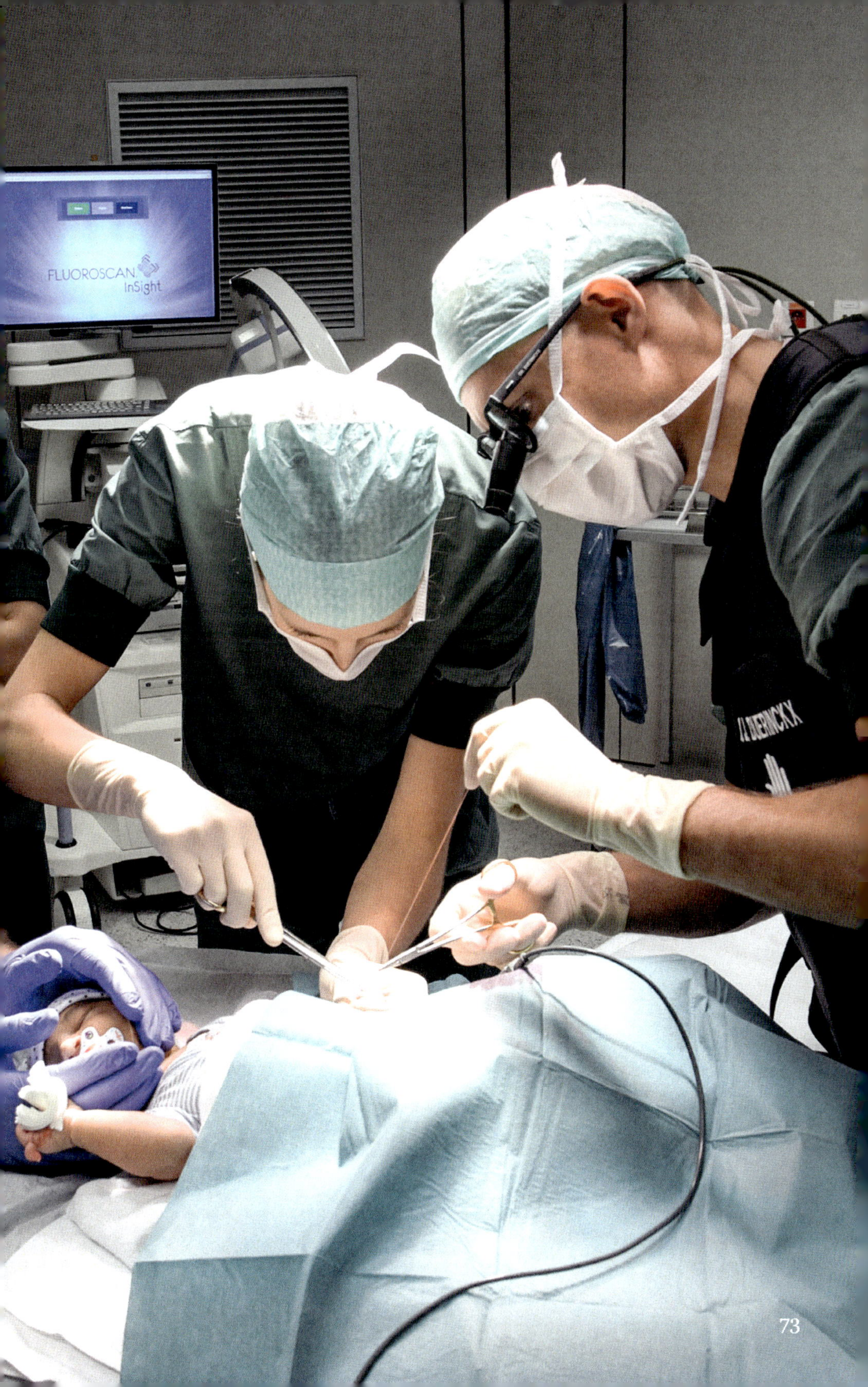
FLUOROSCAN
InSight

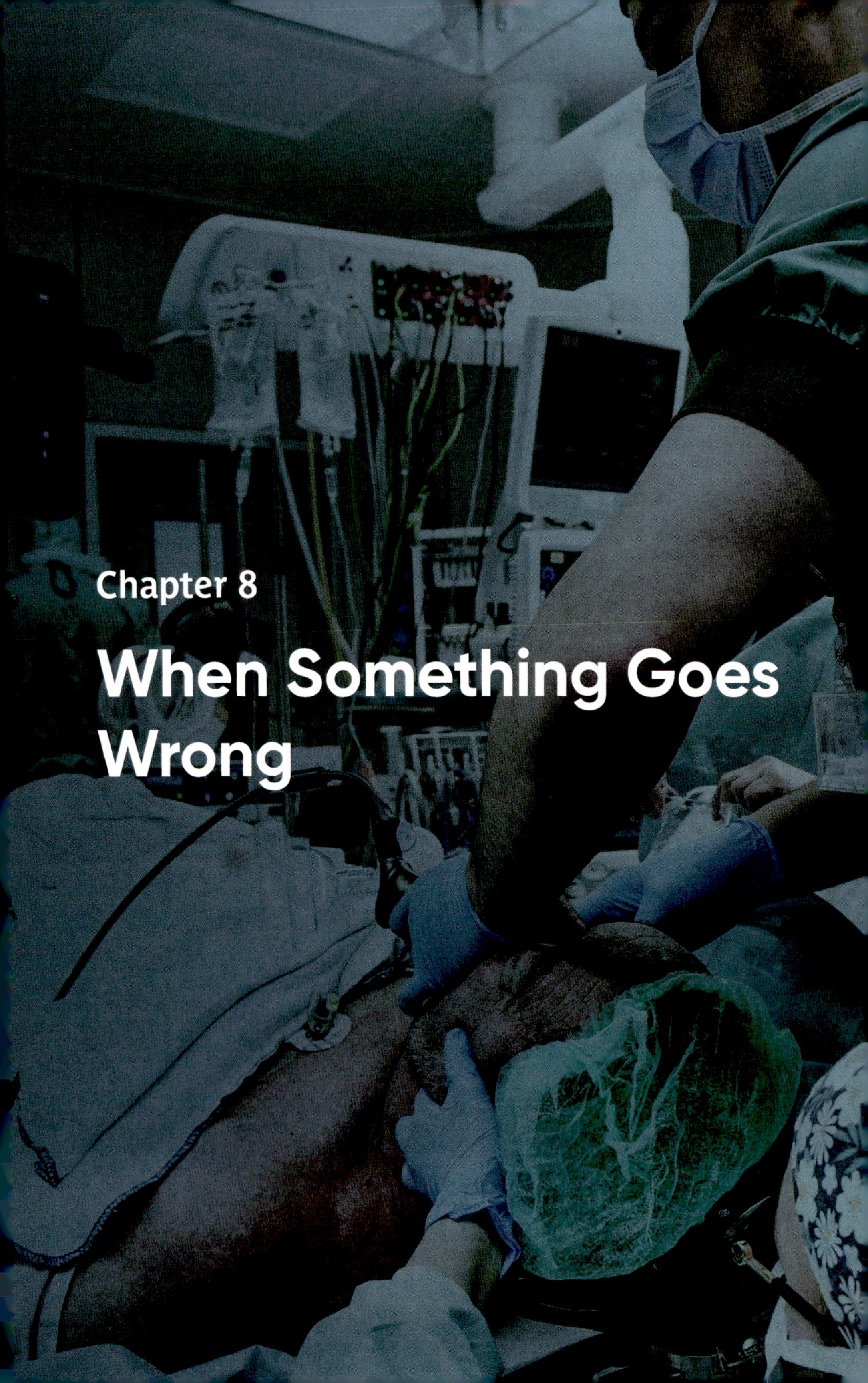

Chapter 8

When Something Goes Wrong

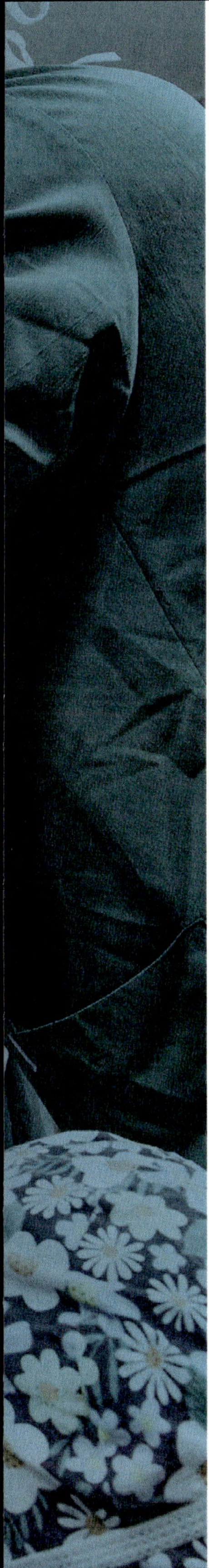

Complications do not arrive with alarms. They arrive quietly, often after you have done everything right.

A loose tooth is disclosed. It is examined. It is documented. The patient is informed. Protective measures are taken. A videolaryngoscope is used. The intubation is careful, deliberate, controlled. And still, the tooth is lost.

From the outside, this is a minor event. From the inside, it lands heavily. You replay the sequence not once, but repeatedly. You know the anatomy. You know the forces involved. You know that the risk was discussed, that consent was informed, that technique was appropriate. And yet the outcome exists. The patient wakes up without a tooth. You are left with the uncomfortable truth that medicine does not reward effort with guarantees.

There is a particular kind of discomfort that comes with these moments. Not panic. Not fear. Something quieter. A tightening in the chest. A slowing of thought.

Some complications stay with you longer.

In 1998, one of my patients developed a peroneal nerve injury after a sciatic nerve block. The result was a foot drop that lasted for months. The nerve block was performed according to the standards of that era. The complication, though rare, was known to occur even in the best of hands. None of that mattered to the patient struggling to lift her foot.

I joined the patient to every physical therapy session. Not as a duty, but because it felt necessary. I watched the exercises. I listened. I asked myself the same question again and again, not whether something could have been done differently, but what, precisely. Needle trajectory? Controlling injection pressure? Better ways of monitoring needle-nerve relationship to prevent the nerve injury?

That complication did not end with full recovery. It followed me into studying the potential causes, into questioning, into research. It changed the way I thought about nerve injury, not as an abstract risk, but as a mechanical and physiologic process that could be better understood, detected earlier, and ultimately prevented.

It set me on a path to study the mechanisms of nerve injury in regional anesthesia. To examine injection pressure as a warning signal rather than an afterthought.

To define electrical nerve stimulation thresholds that reflect needle-nerve proximity before contact occurs, before injury, even when ultrasound appears reassuring. It became clear that safety lies in layered feedback, not in a single technology.

Complications strip away the illusion that experience confers immunity. They teach humility in a way textbooks cannot.

You do not forget these patients. You carry them forward. In how you teach. In how you practice. In the standards you refuse to accept as "good enough".

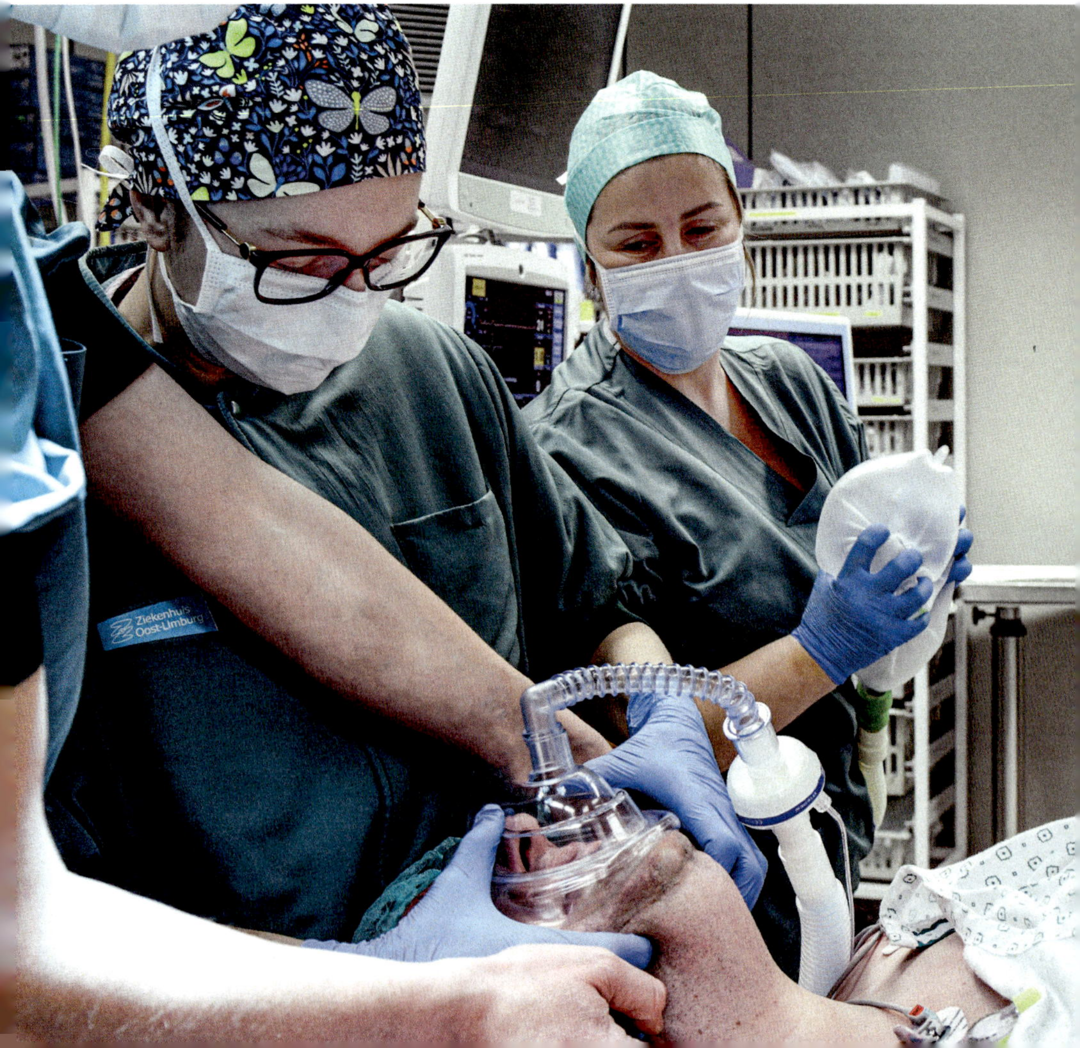

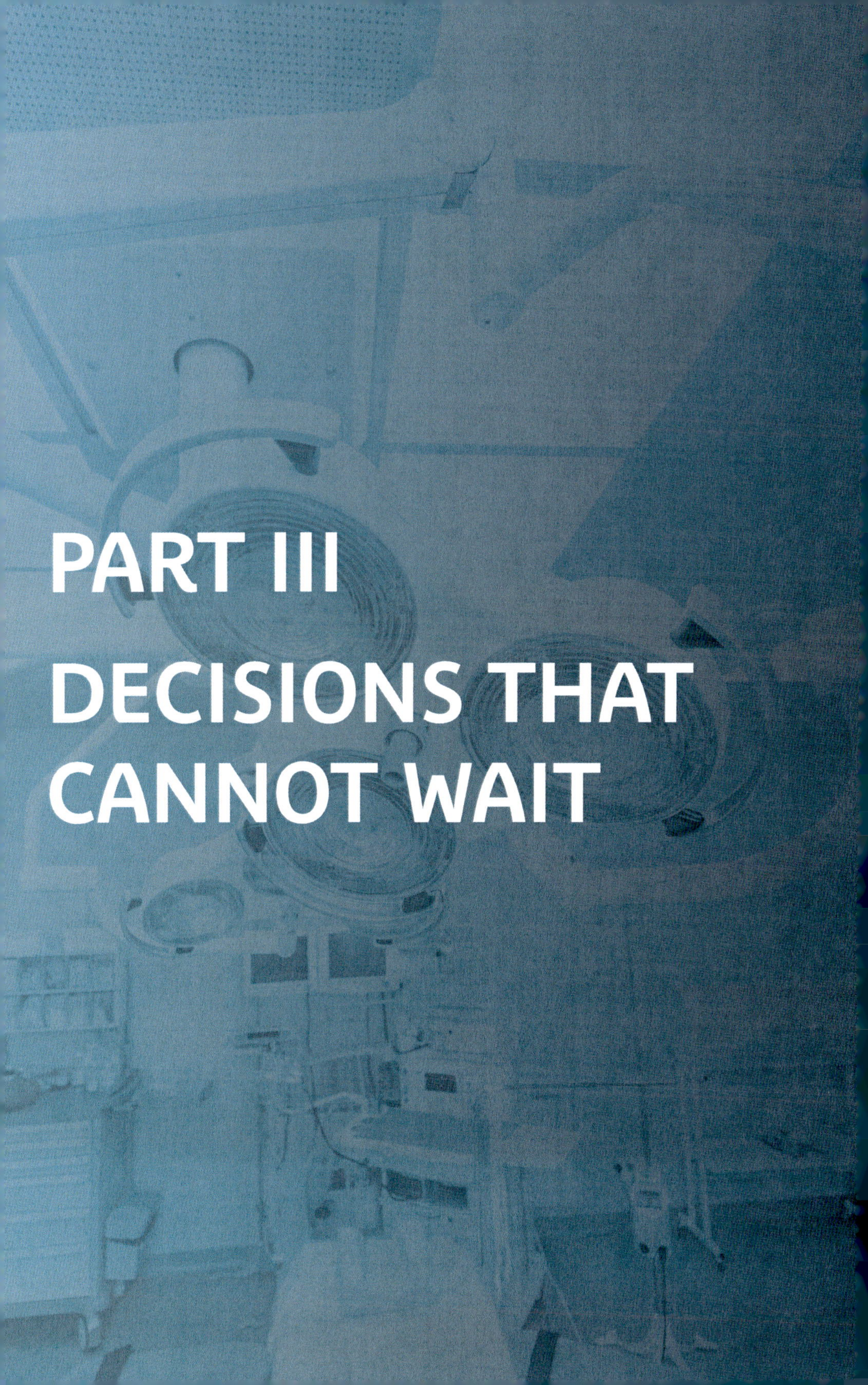

PART III

DECISIONS THAT CANNOT WAIT

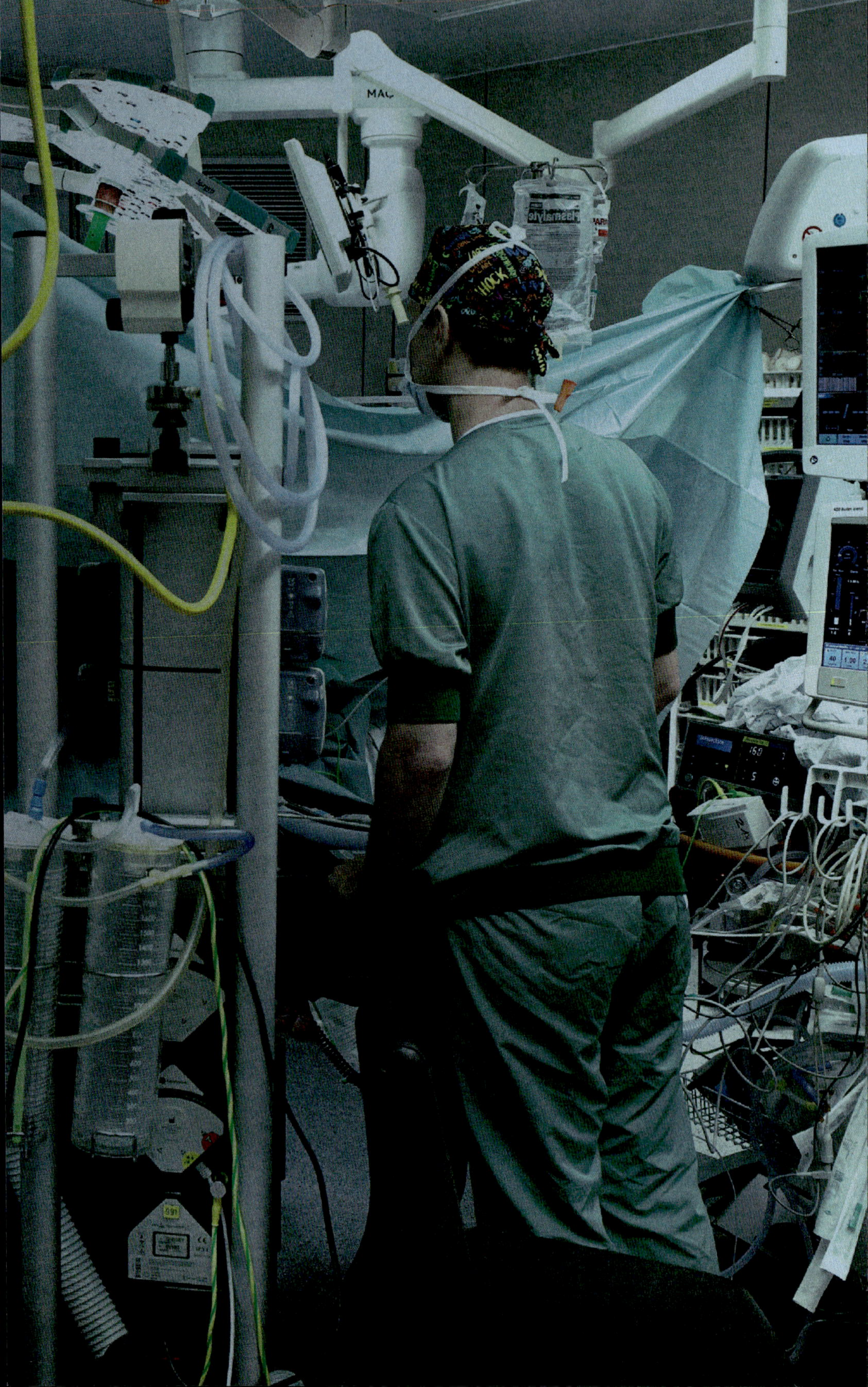

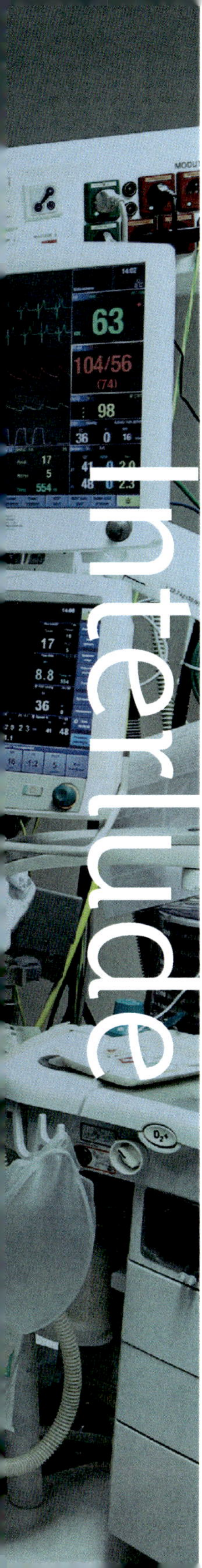

The Myth of Invincibility

From the outside, anesthesiologists can appear fail-safe. We stand at the head of the bed, calm, composed, apparently untouched by urgency or emotion. When physiology wavers, we correct it. When crises emerge, we respond without visible hesitation. To patients, and often to our other specialties colleagues, we seem almost immune to distraction, doubt, or fatigue.

The truth is far more human. Anesthesiologists do not arrive in the operating room unburdened by life. We come to work carrying the same concerns as everyone else. A child with fever at home. A babysitter who cancels at the last minute. A phone call about your aging parent who has fallen and may have broken a hip. Messages unanswered because gloves are already on and the room is ready. On the table lies someone with a ruptured appendix, bleeding internally, septic, afraid, in pain, and dependent on your care. The surgery cannot wait. The physiology is unstable. The responsibility is immediate.

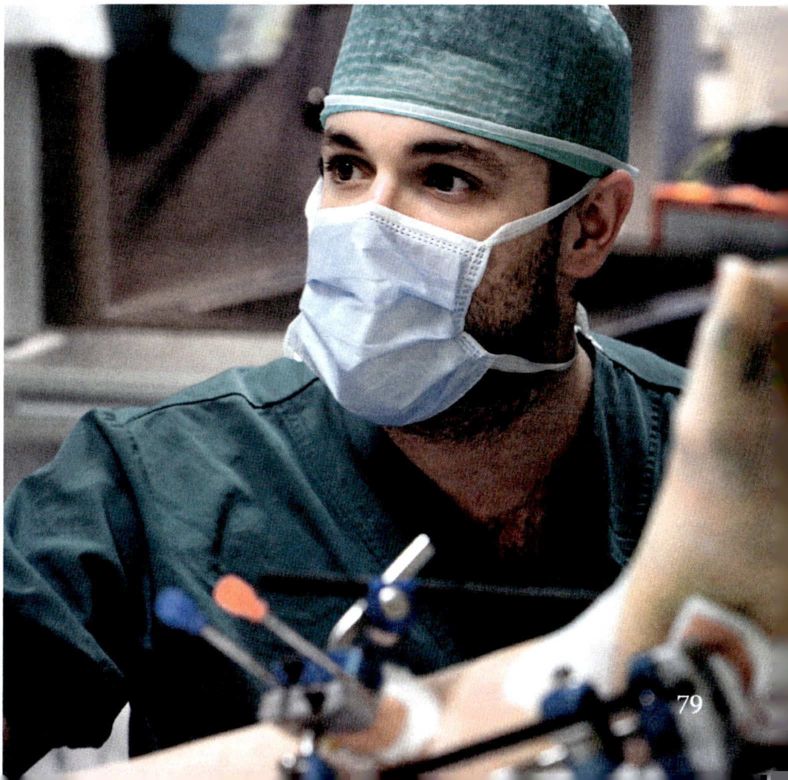

Most professions would allow you to step away. Once the patient is on the table, you stay. You focus. You set everything else aside; because, this matters more, right now. For a time, another human life depends on your presence, your judgment, and your restraint. You cannot leave a patient who depends on you to breathe. You cannot divide attention when a human life is balanced on timing, judgment, and your skills.

So you do something that is never taught explicitly. You learn to manage emotion, not by suppressing it, but by containing it. You learn to postpone fear, concern, and distraction without denying them. You place them carefully to the side, knowing they will still be there later, and you focus on what must be done now.

That is not heroism. It is obligation. A code. And it is what defines the profession of anesthesiology. It is the ability to decide, in real time, what matters immediately and what must wait. It is learning to steer the ship toward safe harbor while the storm continues elsewhere in your life.

Over time, this shapes the way anesthesiologists think and live. You develop an executive mindset; not in the corporate sense, but in the human one.

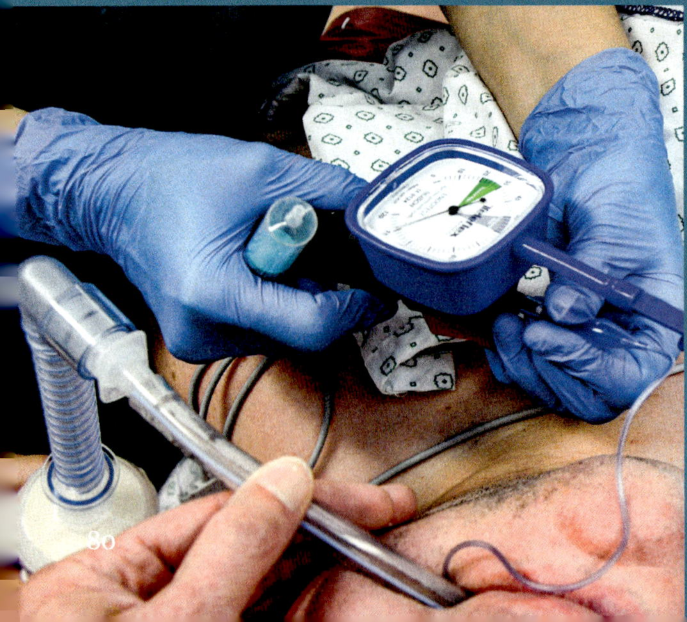

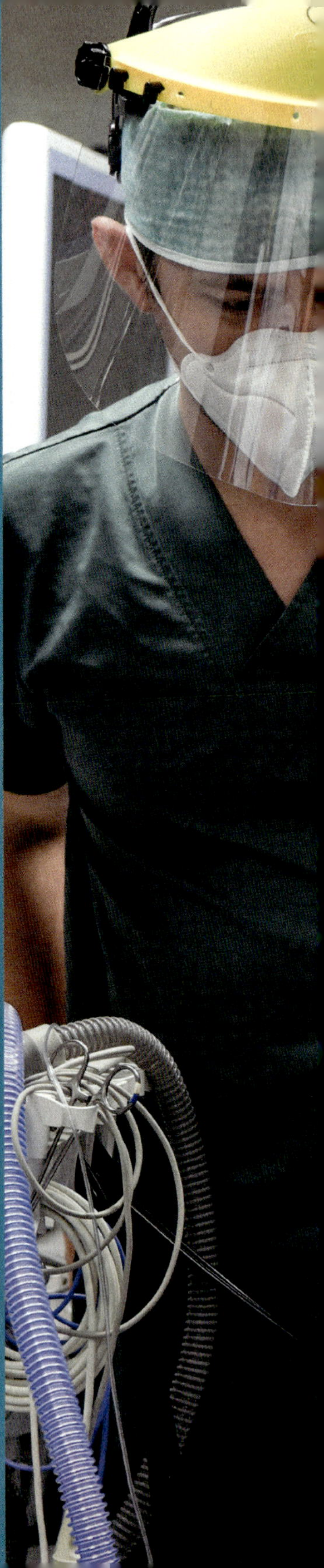

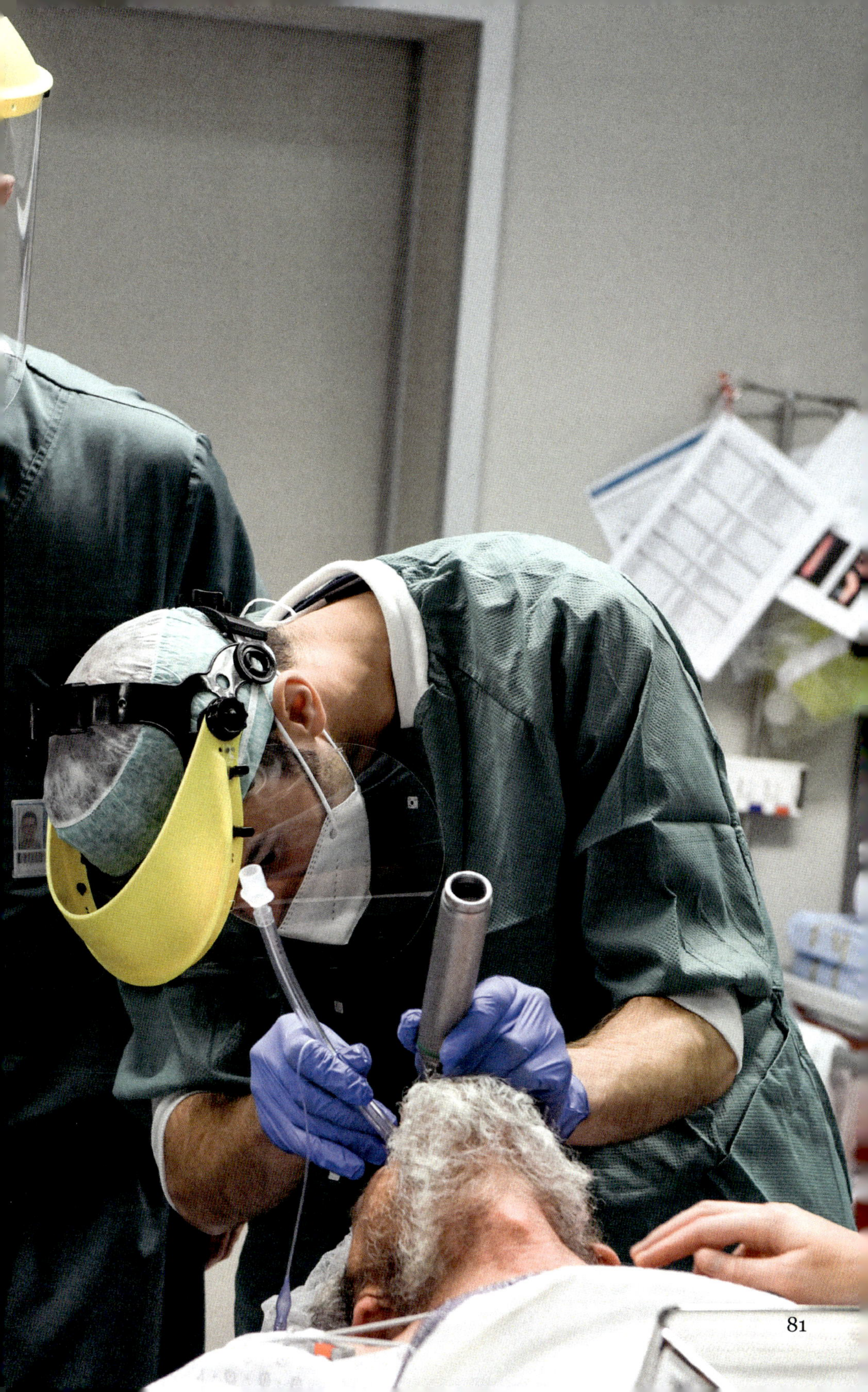

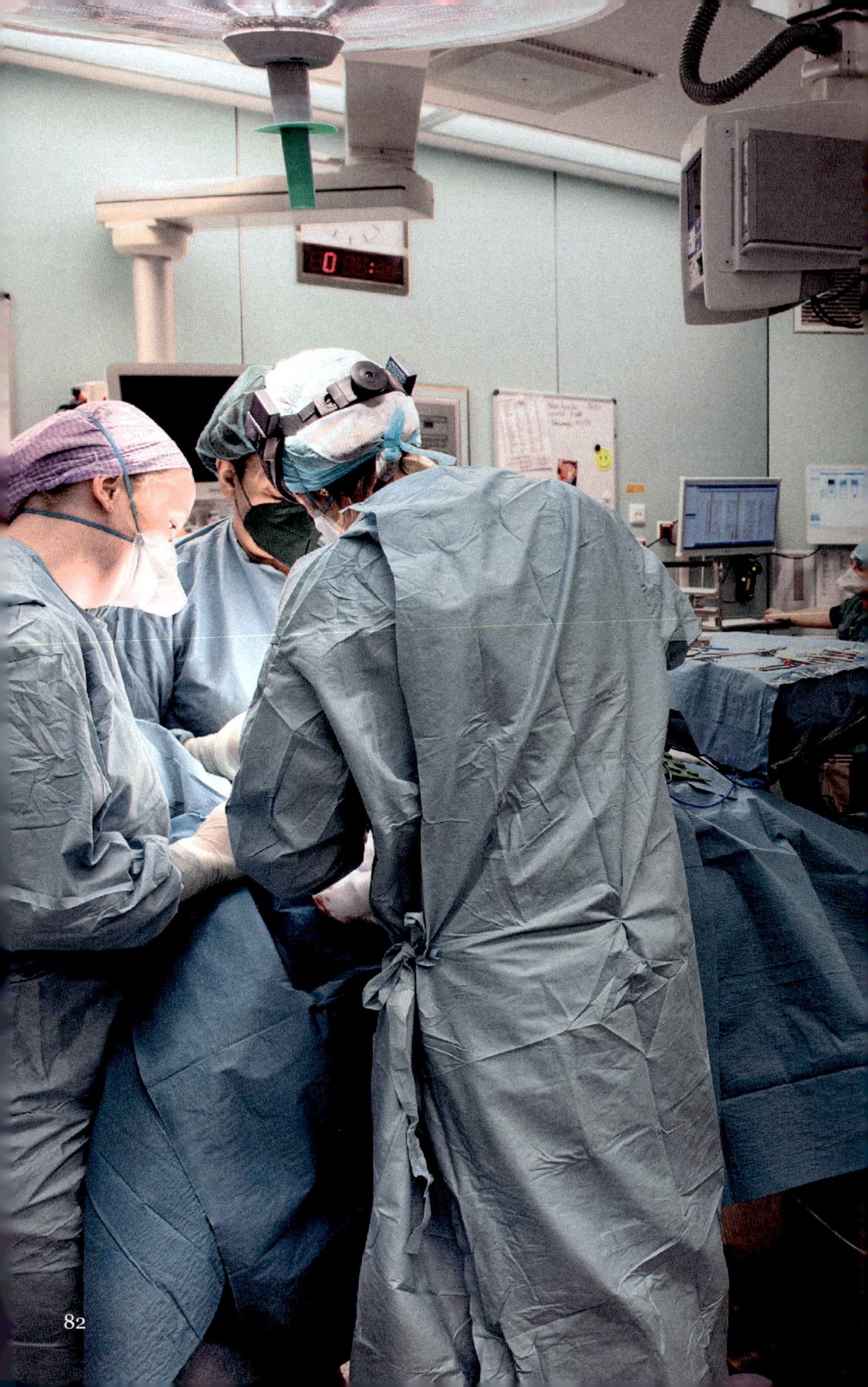

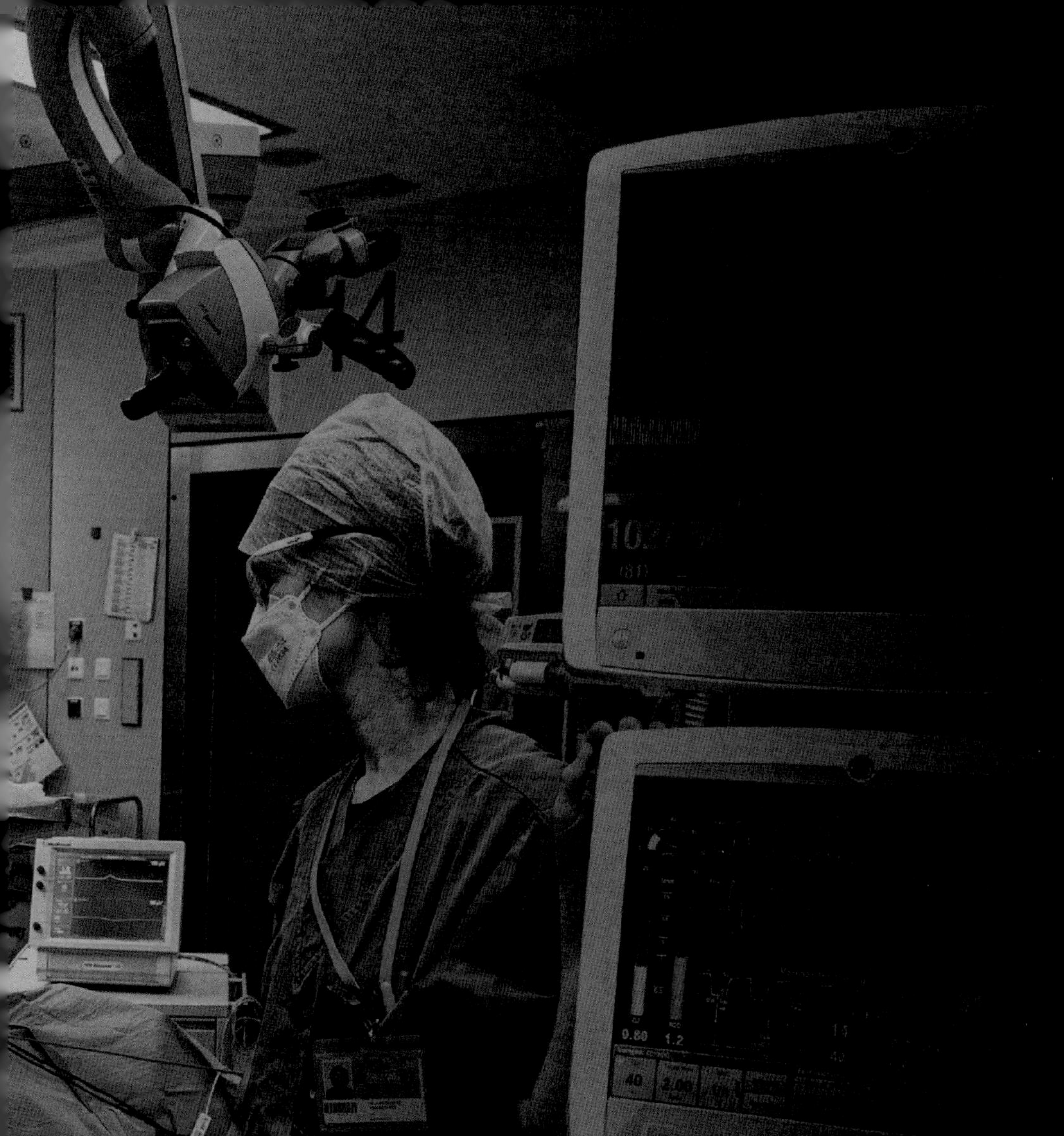

You prioritize without drama. You act decisively without panic. You move forward, even when part of you wants to stop.The calm others see is not the absence of pressure. It is the result of practice in holding responsibility while remaining functional, present, and precise. Practice in carrying the weight of two worlds at once: the one inside the operating room, and the one waiting outside.

When the case is over, when the patient is safe, when the monitors quiet down, only then do you return to what was set aside. Only then do you allow yourself to feel what had to wait.

That discipline, the ability to defer yourself in service of another human being, is what anesthesiology quietly demands.

And that, more than any technique or drug, is what defines the profession.

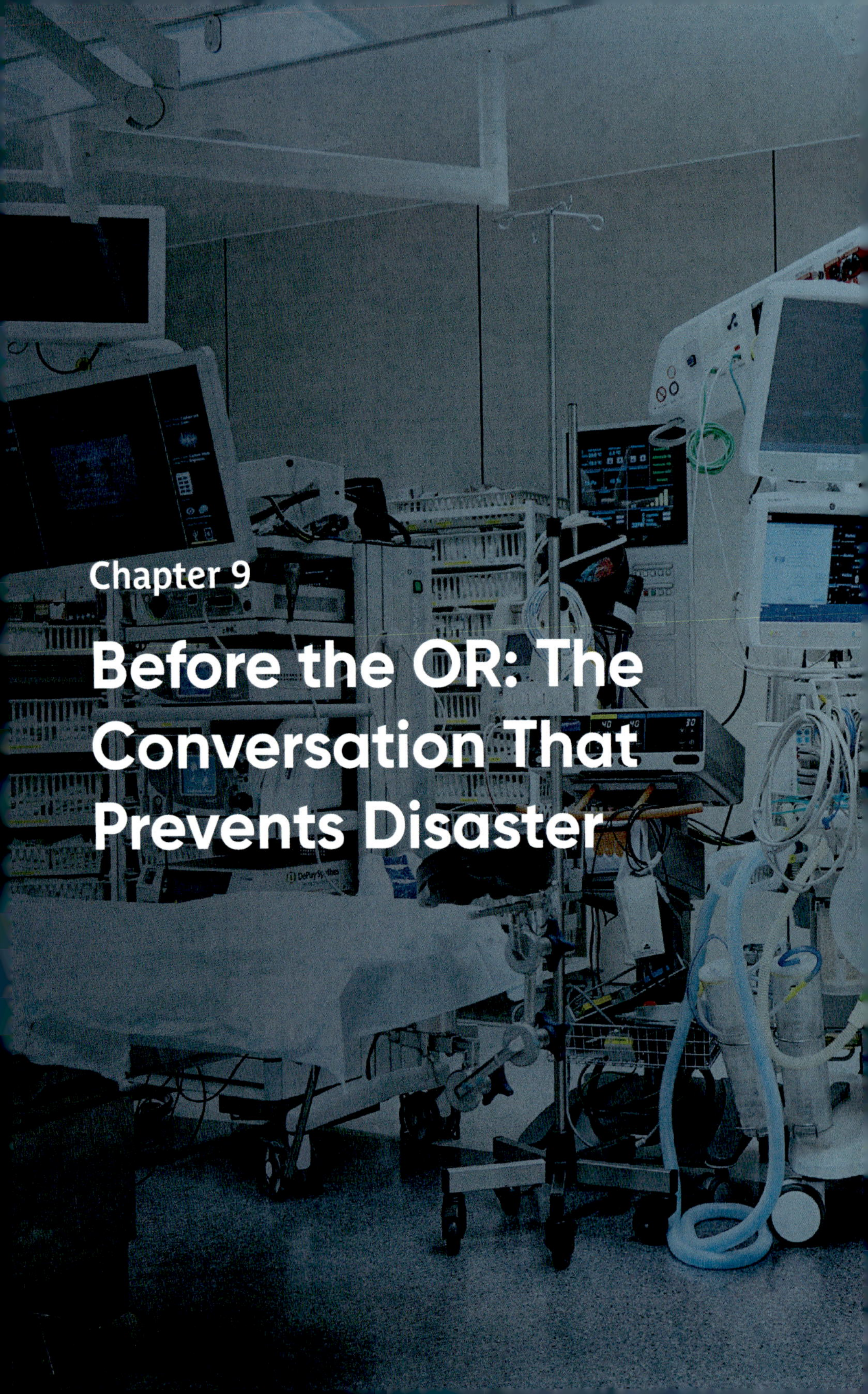

Chapter 9

Before the OR: The Conversation That Prevents Disaster

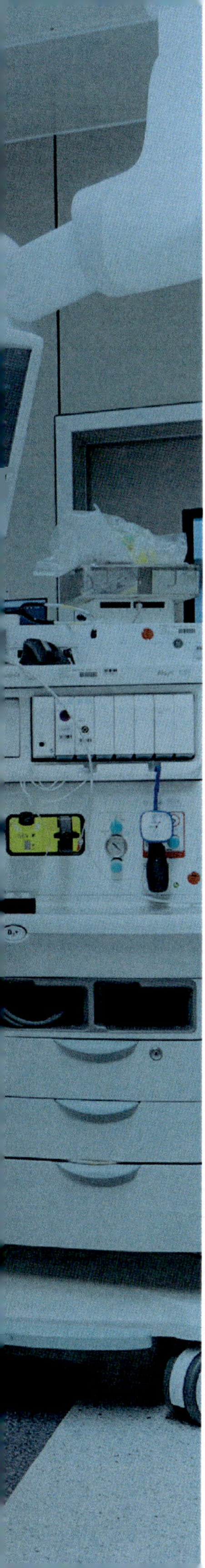

Anesthesia planning does not begin in the operating room. It begins earlier, often days or weeks before, sitting across from a patient who is still fully awake, fully themselves, and quietly trying to understand what is about to happen.

This is where anesthesia strategy and patient trust are built. The preoperative clinic is not dramatic like the operating room. There are no alarms, no bright lights, no urgency in the air. A desk. Two chairs. A chart. Sometimes a computer screen between you and the patient. It looks ordinary, which is precisely why its importance is often underestimated. Yet more crises may be prevented in this room than in an operating theater later.

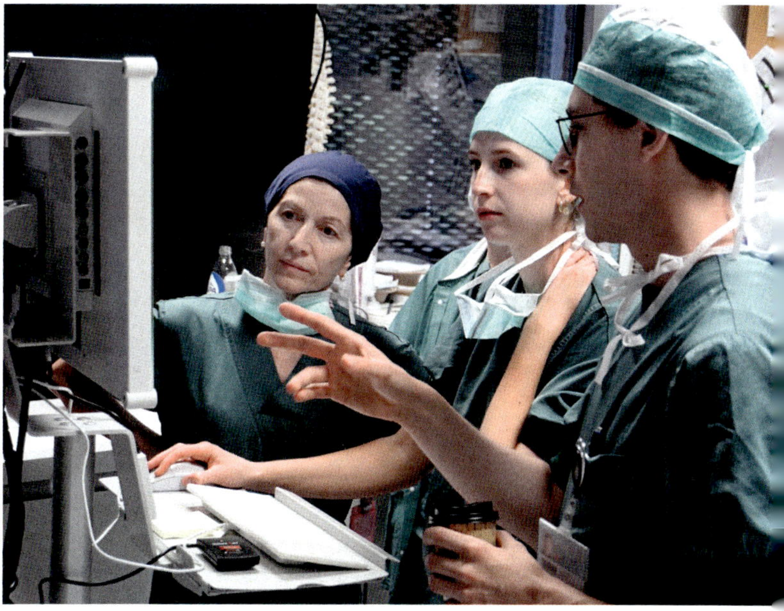

Patients often arrive believing this visit is administrative; a formality before "the real work" happens. They expect questions about allergies, fasting, and medications. They do not understand how much of their outcome is quietly shaped here. This is where we listen for what is not obvious, where small details carry disproportionate weight. Sleep apnea hidden behind a casual mention of snoring.

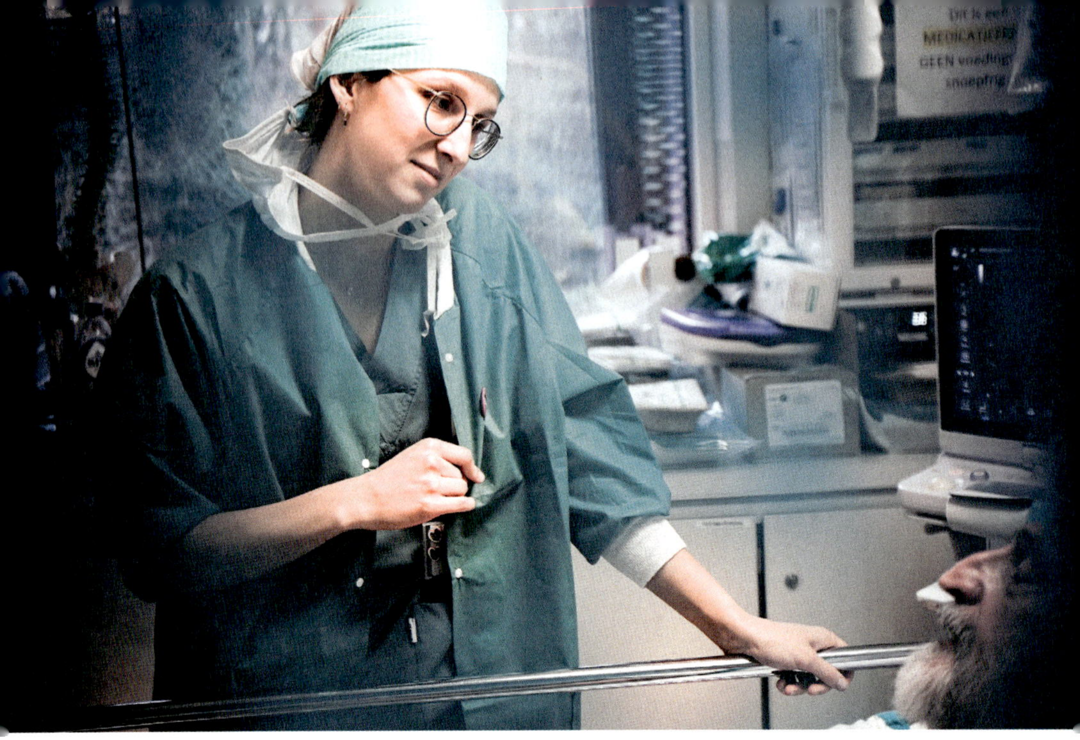

Blood thinners mentioned as an afterthought.

We spot an unsteady gait that contradicts a "healthy" medical file. A past anesthetic experience described vaguely as "not great."

None of these announces itself as a crisis. But together, they form a forecast. Anesthesiology is often compared to aviation and flying a plane. If that is true, the pre-op clinic is weather briefing, fuel calculation, and route planning combined. You do not wait for turbulence to appear at 30,000 feet to decide whether it could matter.

This is where risk is assessed; not as a checklist, but as a narrative. Numbers matter, but context matters more. Age alone does not define risk. Neither does diagnosis. Two patients with the same condition may tolerate anesthesia very differently. Frailty, functional reserve, anxiety, prior trauma, expectations; these are variables that never appear on monitors, yet profoundly shape how physiology behaves under stress.

It is also where rapport is established. Patients rarely remember the pharmacology we explain. They remember how we made them feel. Whether they felt rushed or heard. Whether their fear was dismissed or acknowledged. Whether the person who will take over their breathing seems present, calm, and trustworthy.

We explain what anesthesia will do and what it will not do. We explain risks honestly.

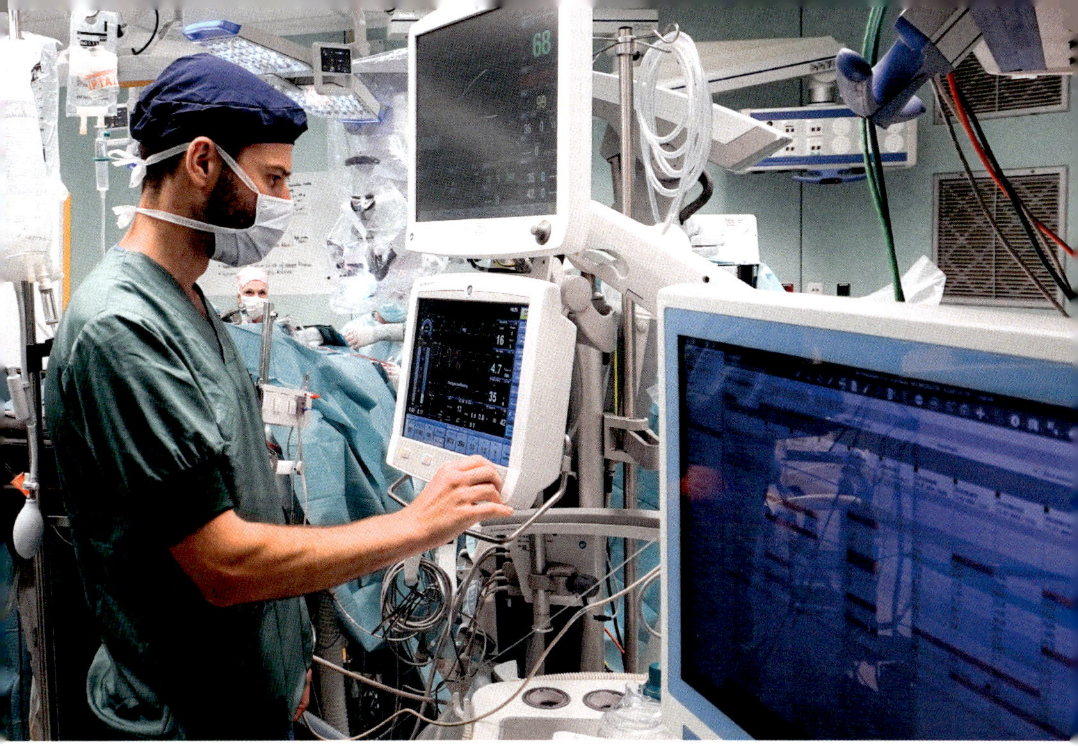

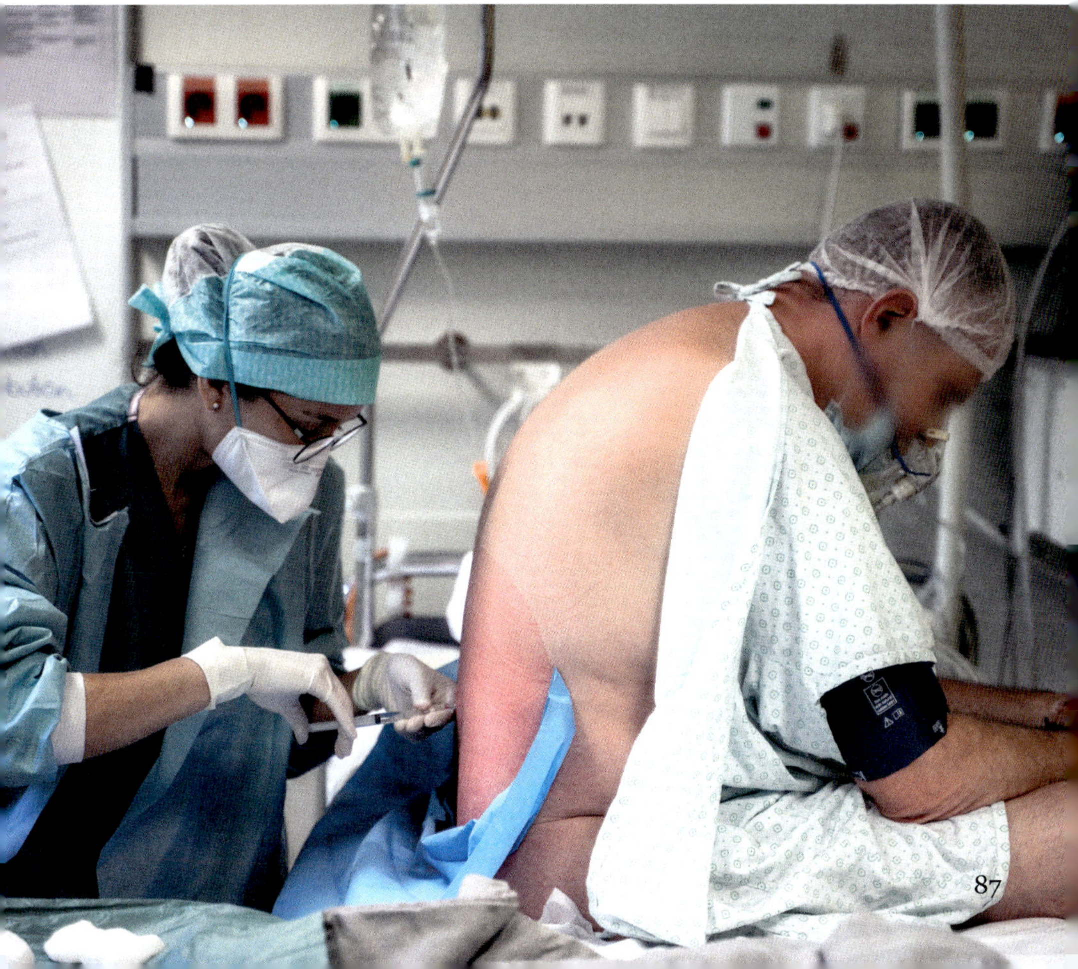

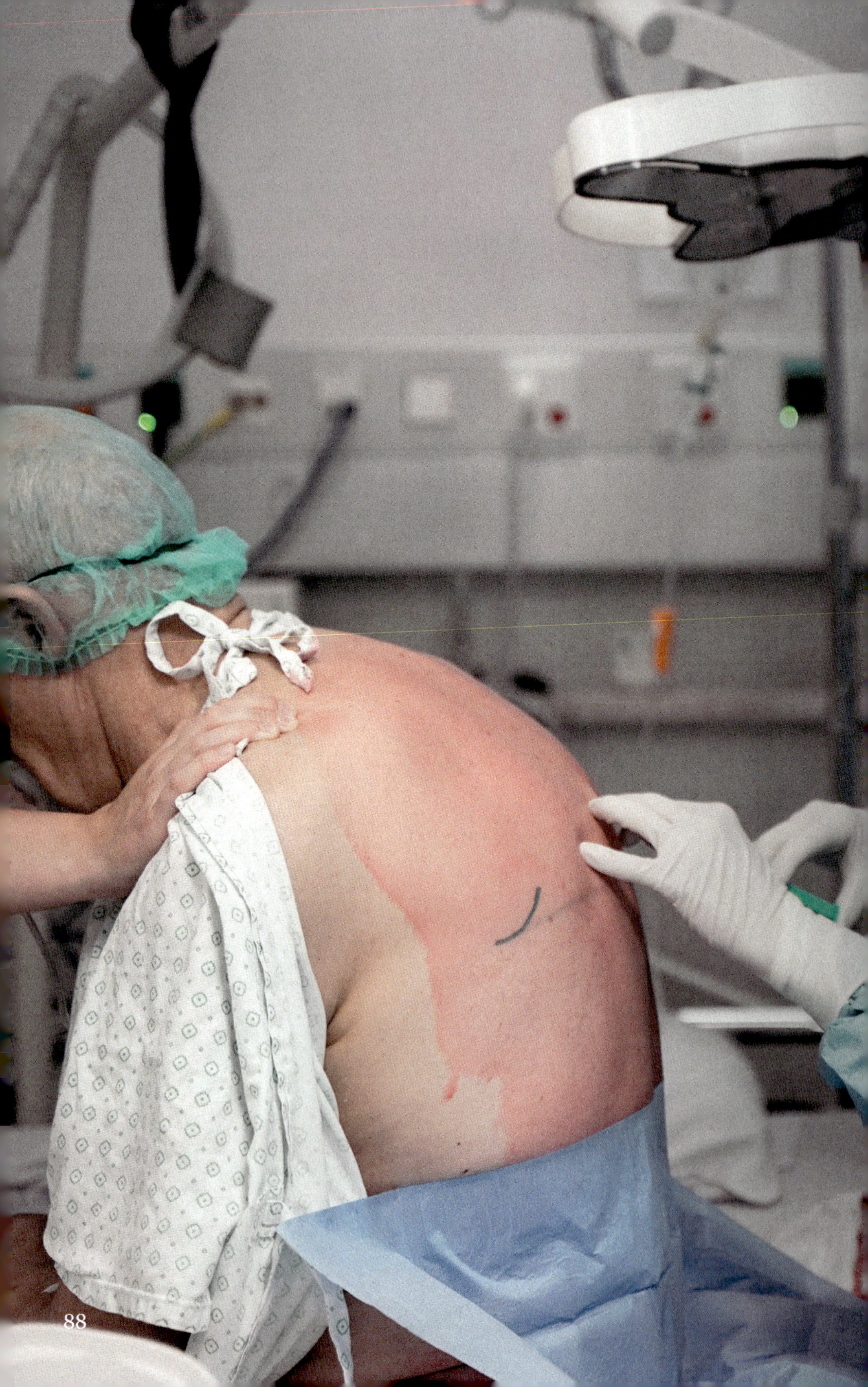

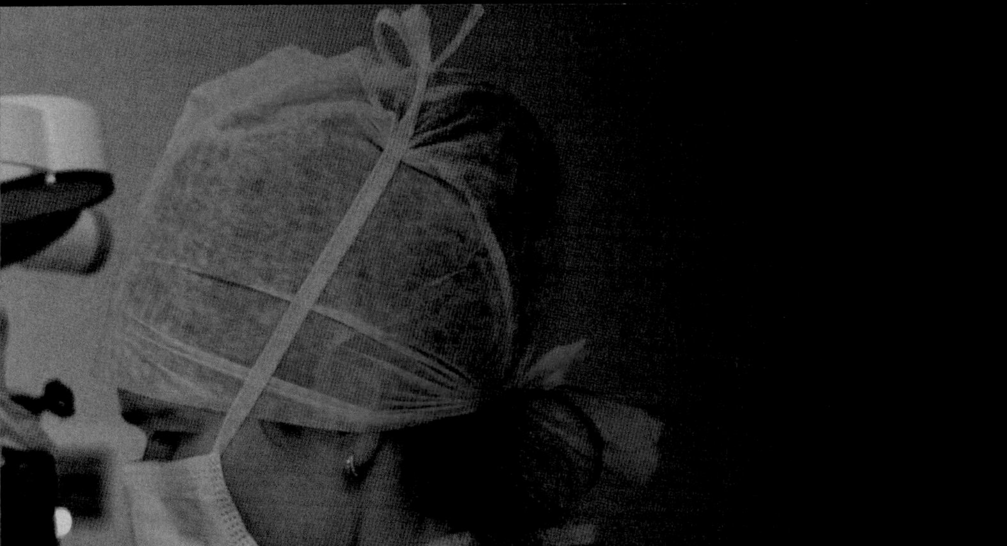

We explain why one technique makes sense over another, not in abstract terms, but in relation to this person, this surgery, this moment in their life. We explain what we will do if things do not go exactly as planned. Not because we expect problems, but because knowing there is a plan is itself reassuring.

Pain control, recovery speed, risk profile, patient preference, surgical requirements, all must align. Consent is not a signature. It is understanding.

Some patients want details. Others want reassurance. Both deserve honesty. Optimization happens quietly here as well. Adjusting medications. Timing anticoagulation appropriately. Flagging untreated sleep apnea. Coordinating with surgeons, cardiologists, internists. Sometimes the most important anesthesia decision is postponing surgery; because the risk today is unnecessary when it can be reduced tomorrow.

The irony is that patients rarely credit anesthesiologists for what never occurred. They will thank the surgeon whose work they can see.

They will praise the nurses who cared for them afterward. The absence of drama rarely earns recognition. They all do deserve the praise. But anesthesiologists know. The preoperative clinic will never make for dramatic photographs. But it is one of the most powerful rooms in perioperative medicine. It is where anesthesiology shows its true character: thoughtful, deliberate, human.

Long before the monitors begin to beep, anesthesia has already begun, quietly, with a conversation meant to ensure that nothing extraordinary needs to happen later.

And when nothing does, that is not luck. That is our work in the preop clinic.

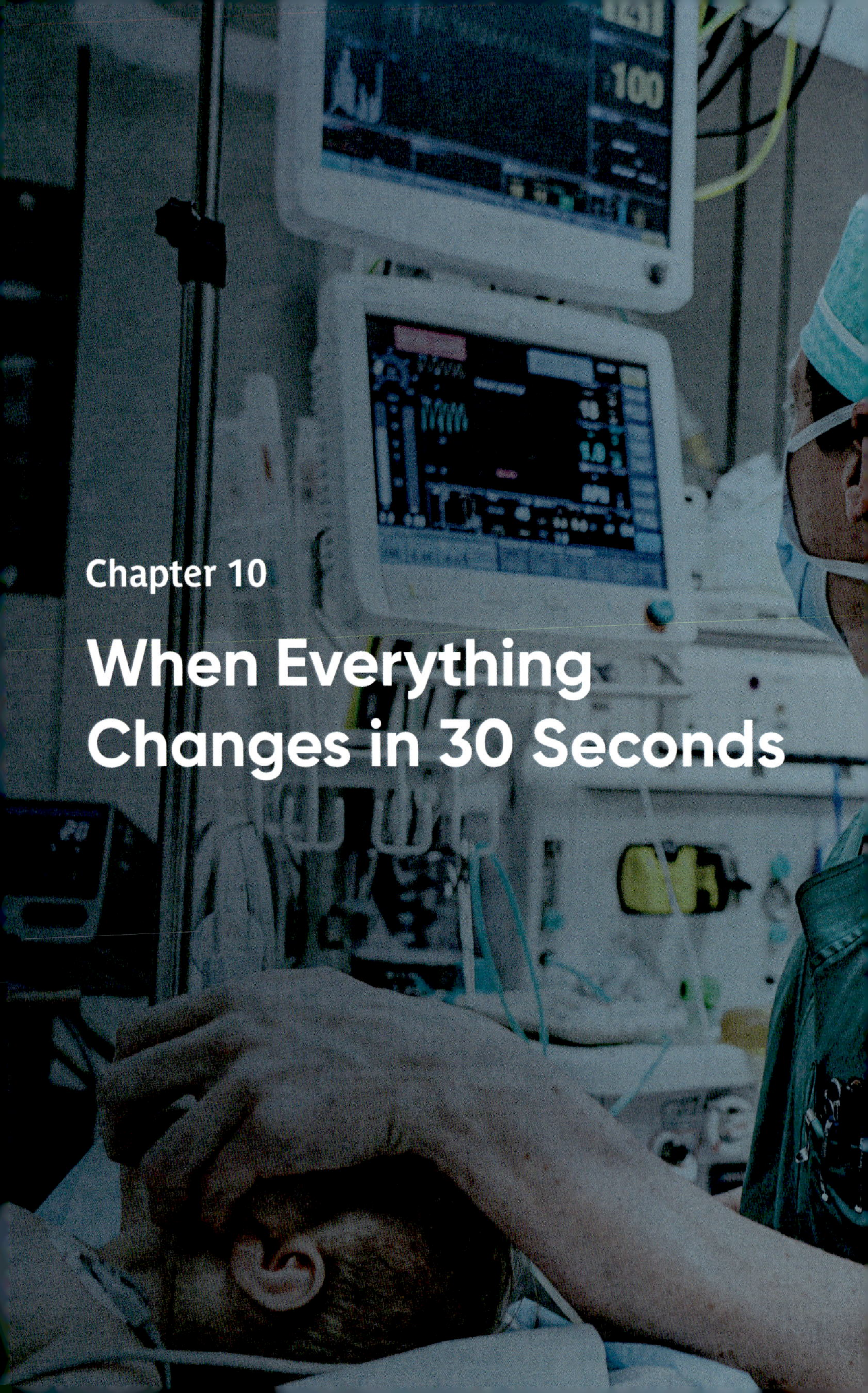

Chapter 10

When Everything Changes in 30 Seconds

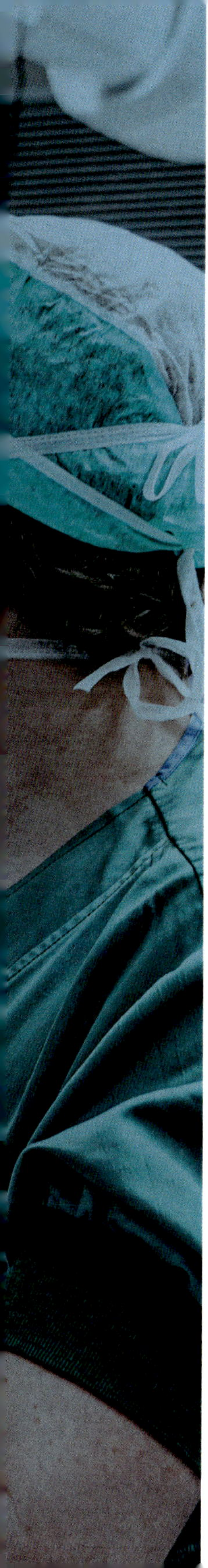

Most anesthetics unfold quietly. Monitors trace predictable patterns. Mechanical ventilation via breathing machine is steady. Blood pressure drifts within acceptable limits. The room settles into a rhythm that feels almost repetitive. This is what people imagine anesthesia to be: calm, controlled, uneventful. And then, sometimes, all of a sudden everything changes.

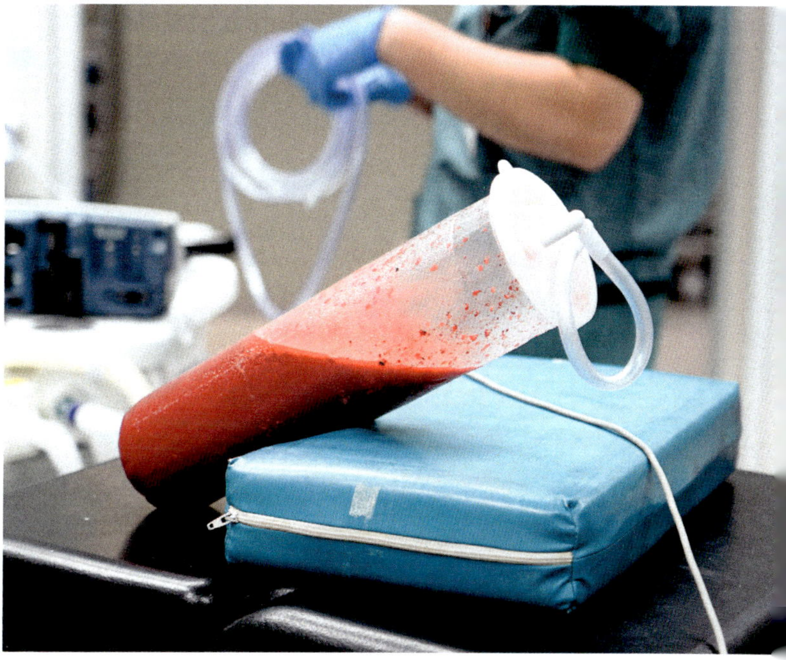

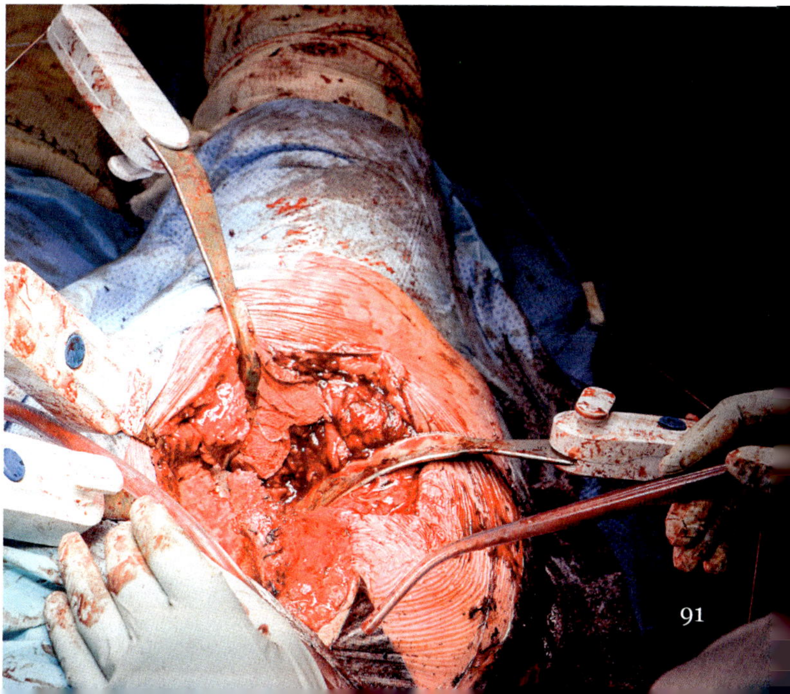

Not gradually. Not politely. But unexpectedly and violently. There may be no warning. No slow buildup. One second the physiology is stable; the next, it collapses. The transition can take seconds.

A routine case in a peripheral hospital. The day in the OR started like another day in the office. Induction uneventful. The airway secure. Ventilation normal. Prophylactic antibiotic was administered, something used countless times before, something no one in the room questioned. But this time the blood pressure vanished. Not drifted. Not dipped. Disappeared. The pulse oximeter struggled to find a signal. The end-tidal CO_2 narrowed abruptly. Ventilation became more difficult as airway pressures climbed. The patient's skin, moments ago warm and pink, turned pale, then mottled.

There is no time to confirm. No luxury of differential diagnosis. In anesthesiology, you are taught this early and repeatedly: when everything fails at once, treat first, analyze later. Anaphylaxis was suspected. And anaphylaxis does not ask for permission.

Administer: Epinephrine. Oxygen. Fluids. Now.

The room changed, not into chaos, but into focus. Emergency resuscitation button was pressed. Colleagues rushed in to help. Orders became short. Movements became deliberate. Someone stopped the suspected trigger, antiobiotic was stopped. Someone opened fluids wide. Someone reached for potent vasopressors without being told. Leadership is rarely louder in a crisis; it is quieter, clearer. This is where preparation reveals itself.

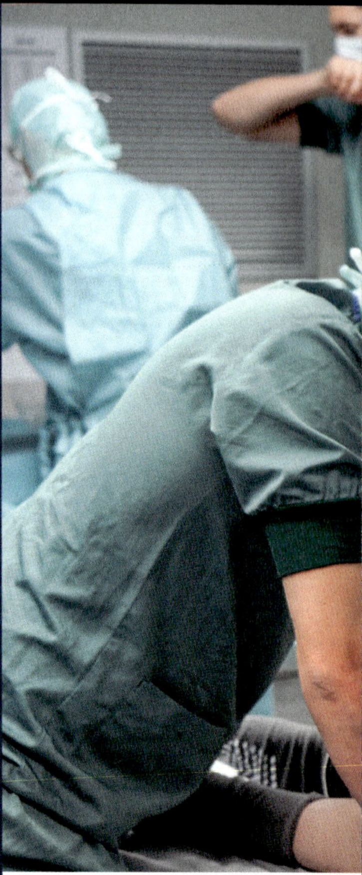

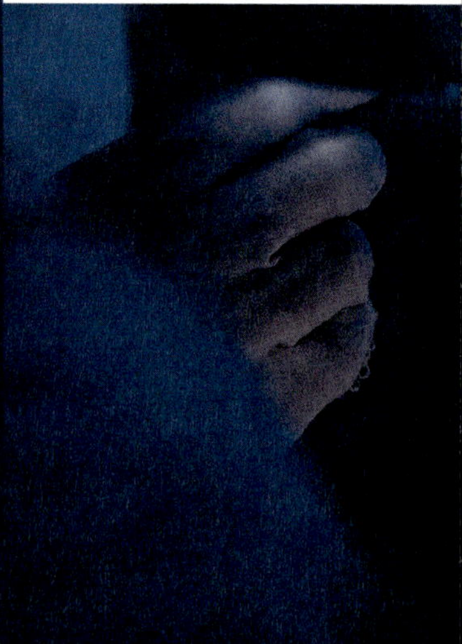

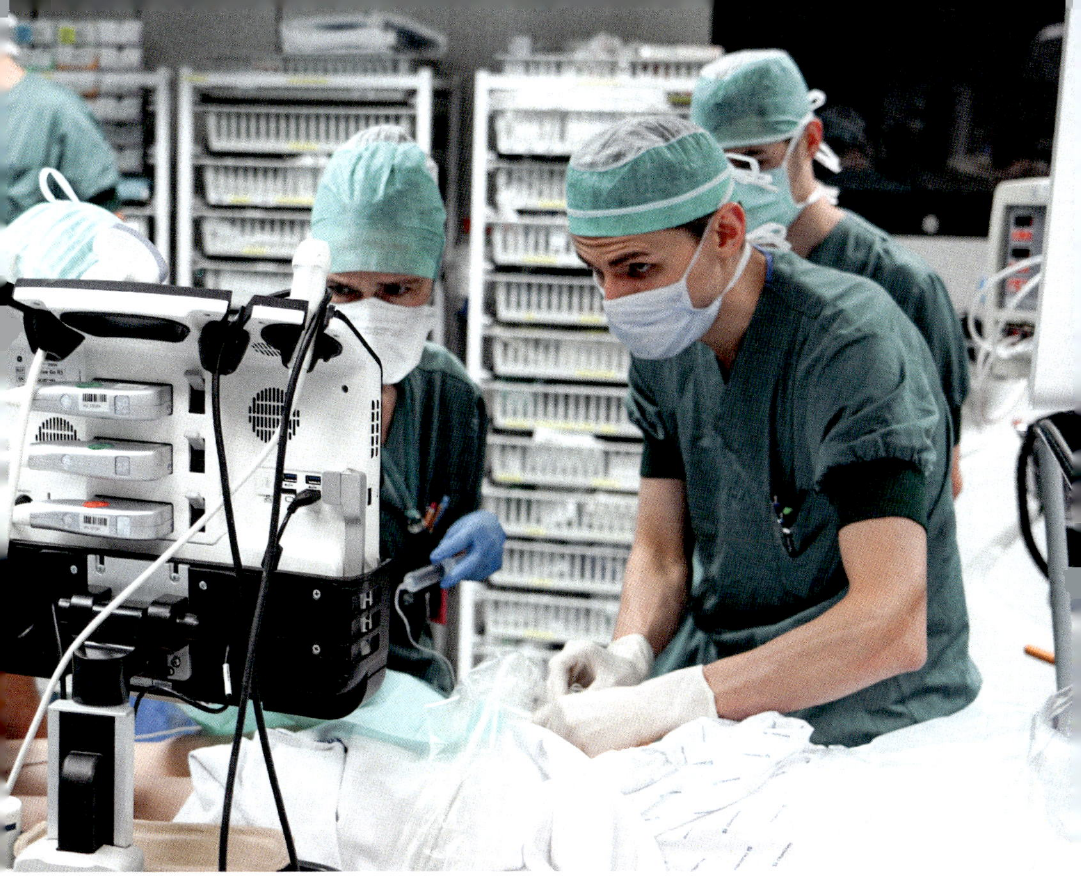

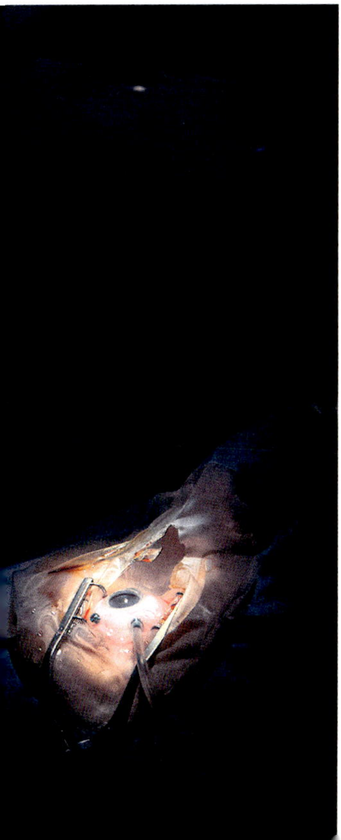

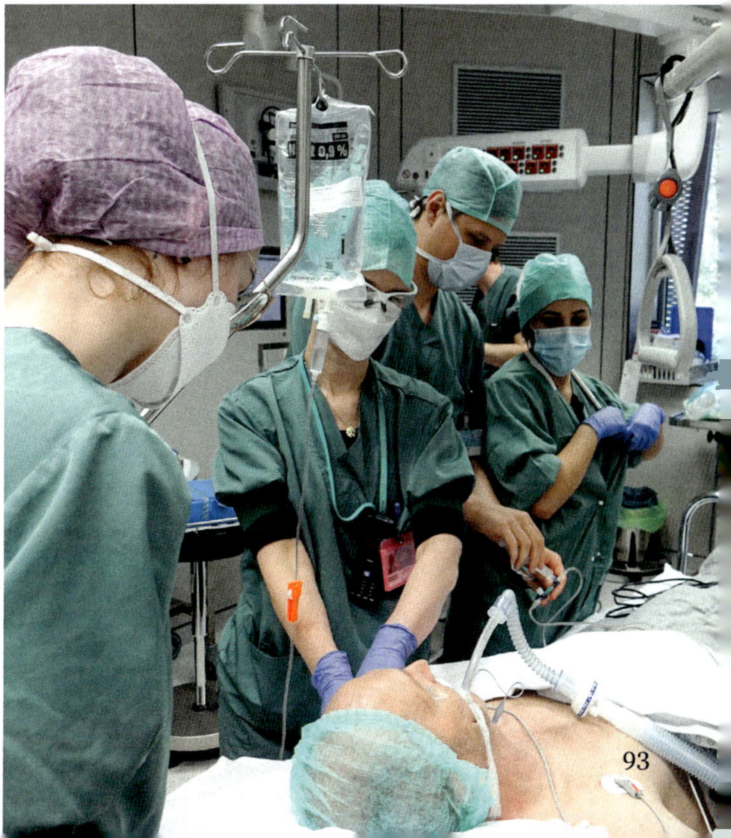
0,9 %

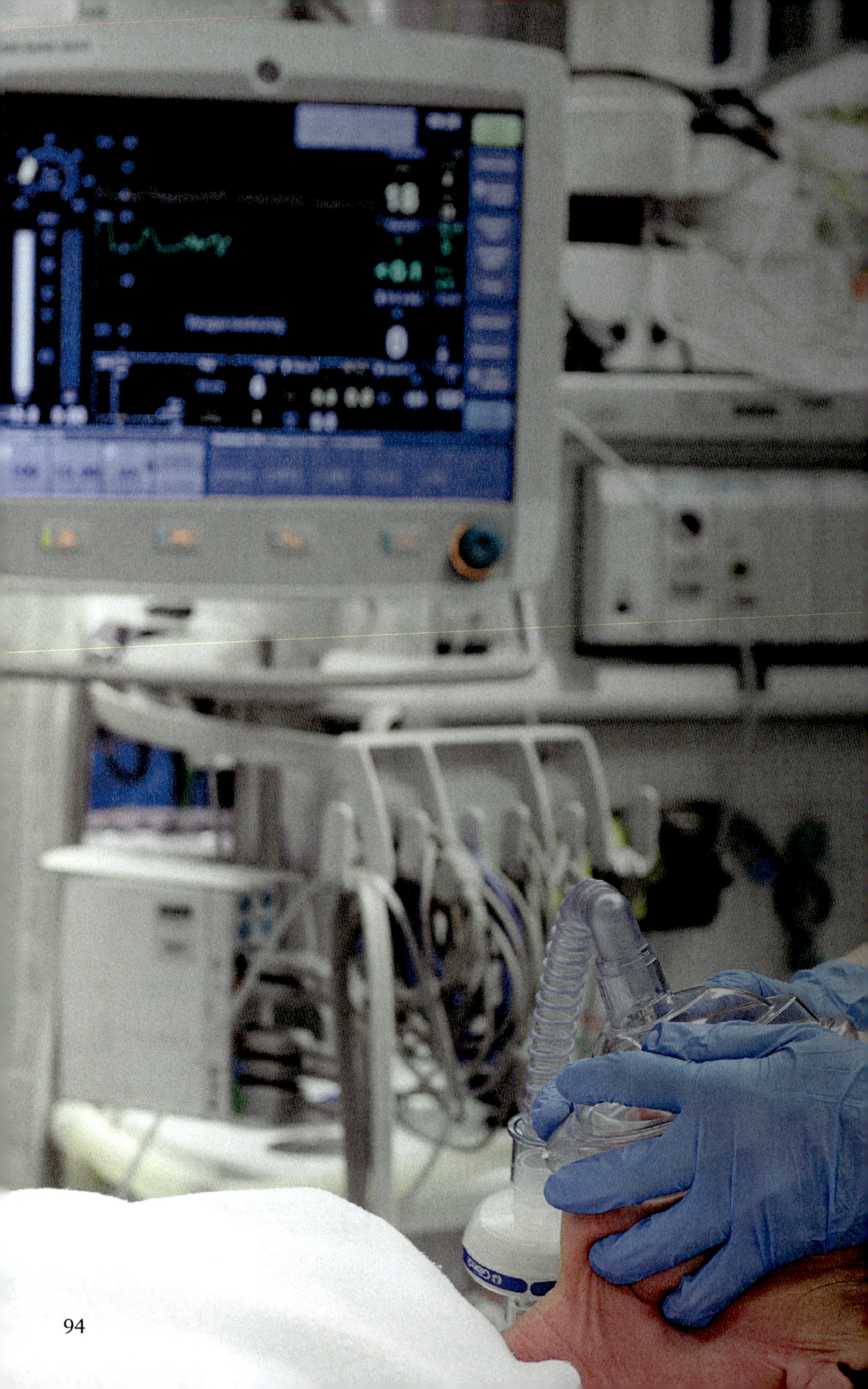

The physiology tells you the truth before the monitors or lab work catch up. You feel it before you can name it.Blood pressure returned in steps, not all at once. Ventilation eased. End-tidal CO_2 widened. Color returned slowly, as if the body were deciding whether it trusted us again.

From the outside, it may have looked controlled. Professional. Almost routine. From inside the anesthesiologist's mind, time had compressed. Thirty seconds felt both instant and endless. Every action mattered. Every delay would have mattered more.

The patient survived. He woke up later, confused but intact. He asked the same questions patients always ask: "Is it over?" "Did everything go okay?" The honest answer was - yes. The complete answer was a lot more complicated.

I remember another case during what was supposed to be a routine cataract surgery, a type procedure often debated as not needing an anesthesiologist in the room. Moments after the surgeon applied standard intraocular drops, the patient suddenly lost blood pressure and pulse.

We immediately activated. The rescue alarm was activated, and within moments, anesthesiologists and nurses filled the room. Emergency medications were given, the patient was intubated, and resuscitation began. A bedside cardiac ultrasound was performed within minutes to differentiate anaphylaxis from a myocardial infarction, both possible in a 70 - year - old with multiple comorbidities undergoing even a minor procedure like cataract surgery.

Anaphylaxis or sudden, massive intraoperative blood loss are some of those moments that strips anesthesiology down to its core. There is no finesse. No elegance. Only recognition, decisiveness, and speed. You do not save a life by being clever. You save it by being prepared.

And when circulation returns, when oxygenation stabilizes, when the storm recedes, nothing about it looks heroic. There is no visible scar. No memory. No sign that the body came dangerously close to its limits. That is the paradox of anesthesiology.

The more serious the crisis, the less the patient will ever know about it. These are reminders that modern anesthesia is safe not because nothing ever goes wrong, but because someone is always ready for the moment it does.

When people call anesthesiologists life savers, they imagine drama. What they don't see is preparation, the quiet discipline that turns thirty catastrophic seconds into a survivable story. After the room resets, after the monitors settle back into familiar rhythms, after the adrenaline fades, the weight arrives, not as fear, but as respect. Respect for how little margin exists.

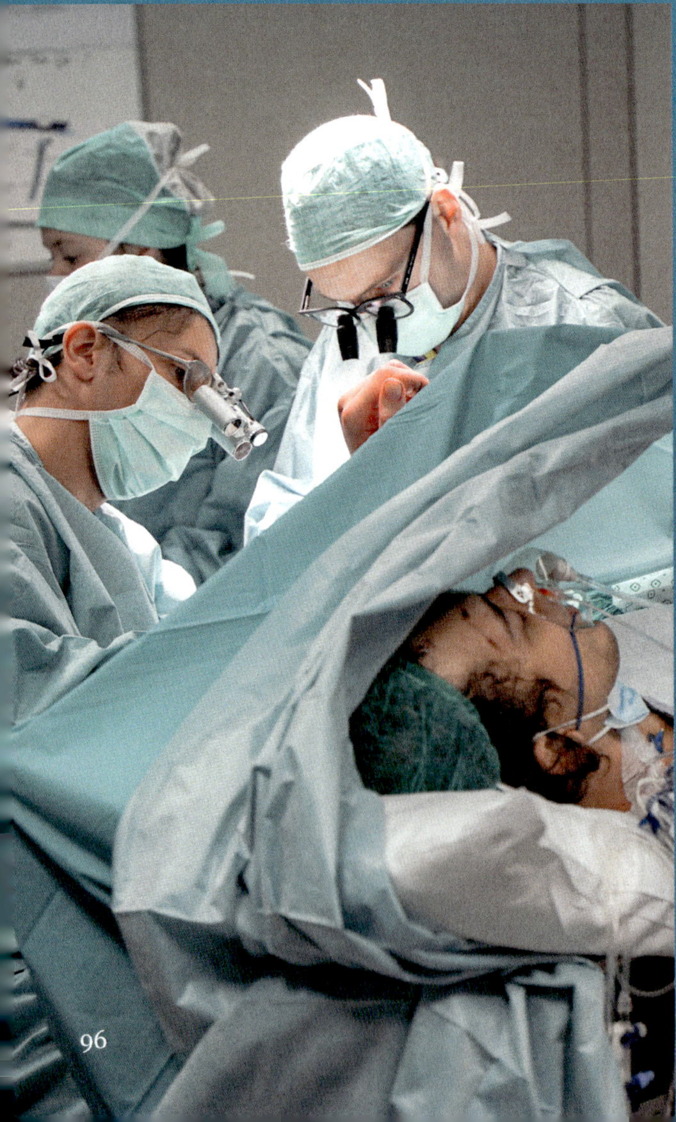

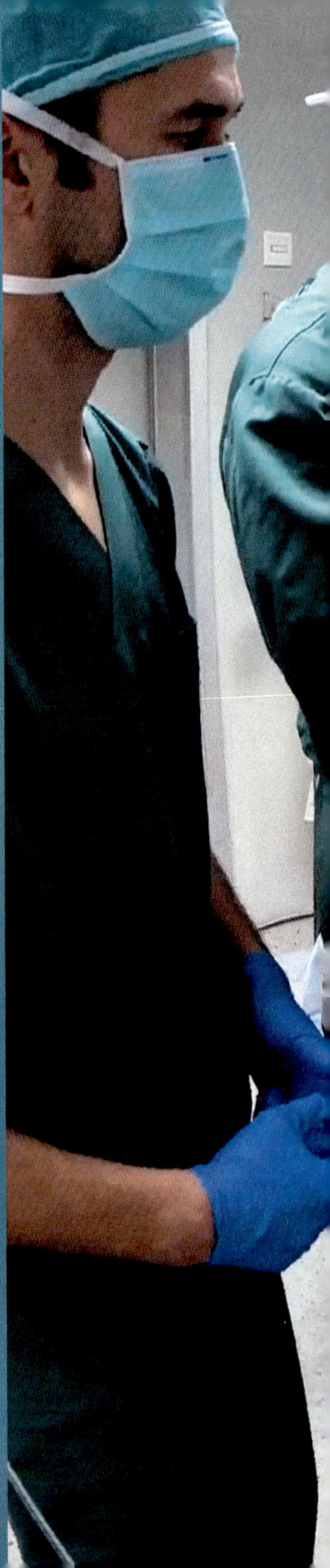

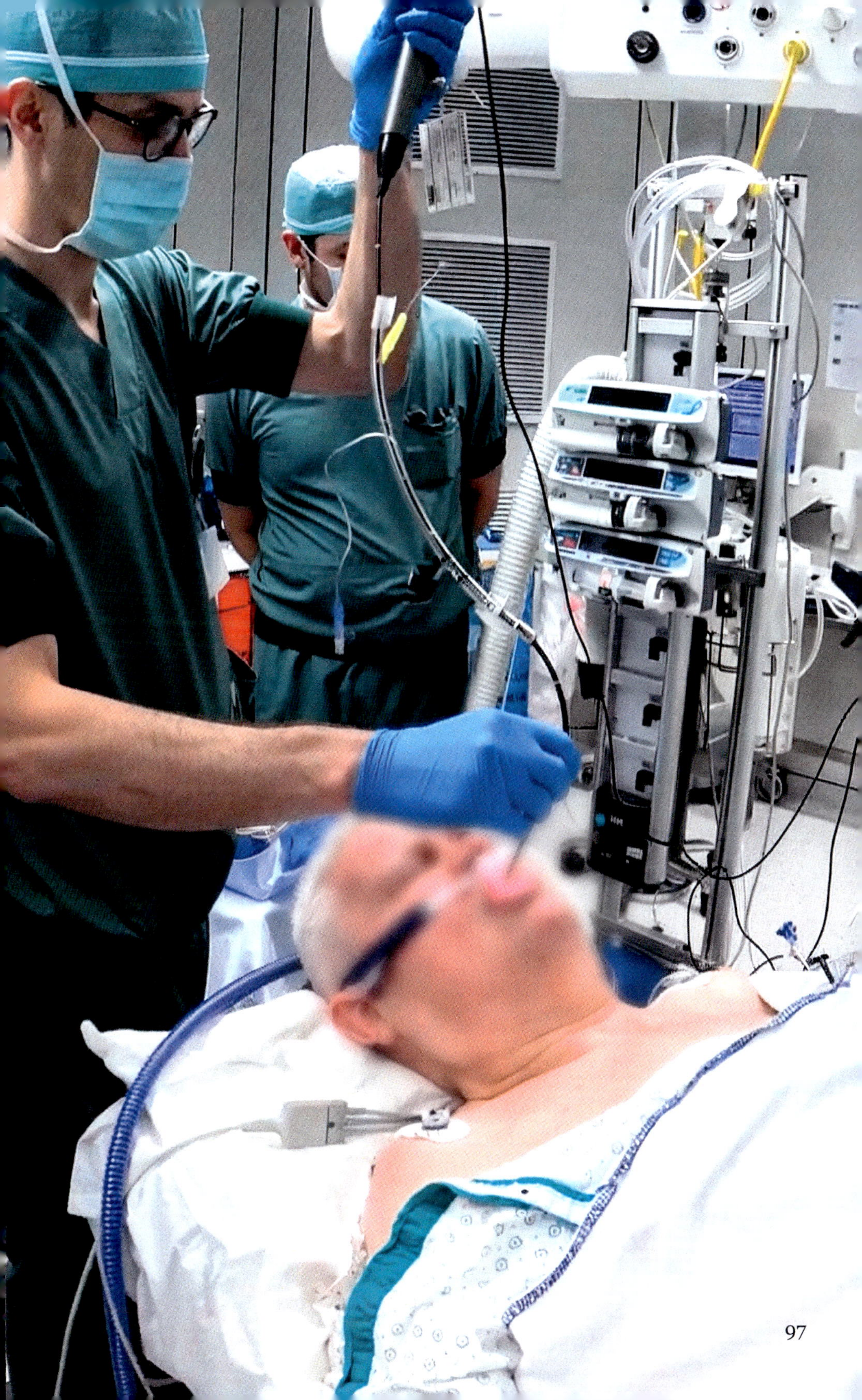

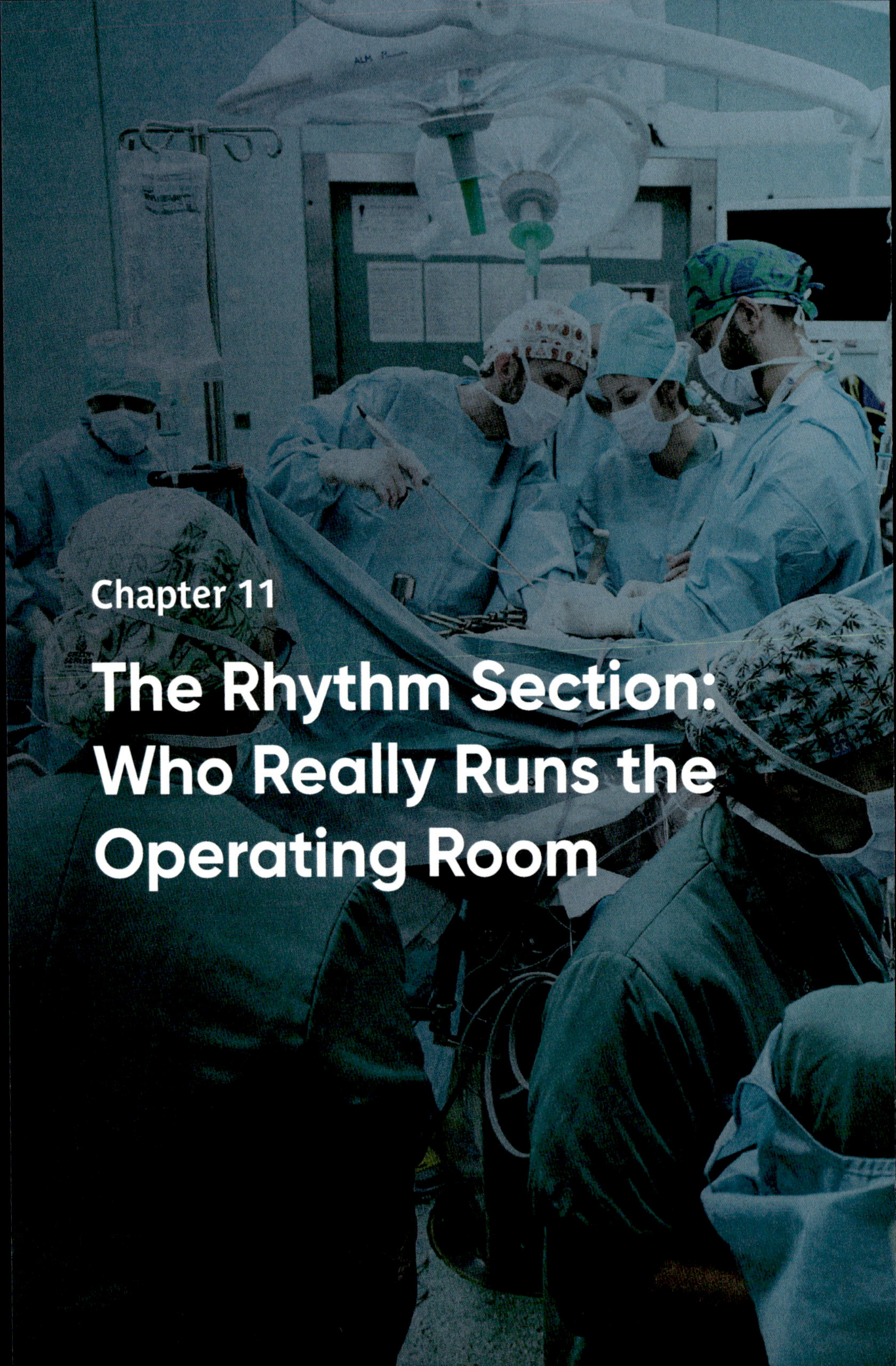

Chapter 11

The Rhythm Section: Who Really Runs the Operating Room

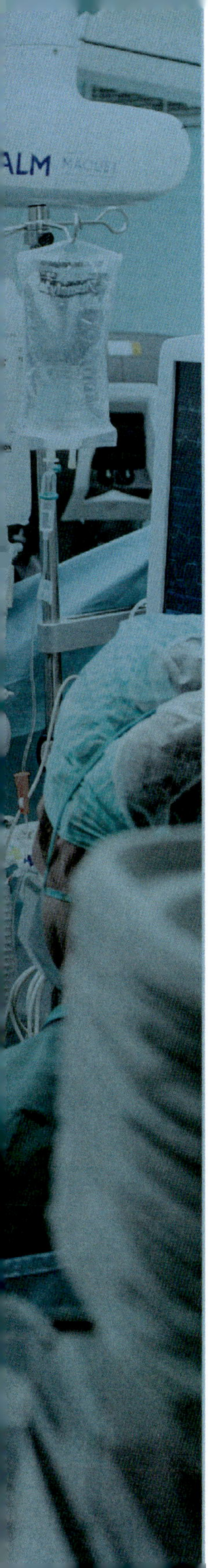

I have often said that anesthesiologists are the rhythm section of the operating room. Not the headline act. The bass and drums, that no one applauds directly, yet everything depends on. Having played bass guitar in touring rock bands, I know that if the rhythm is steady, the music holds together. If it falters, nothing sounds or works right.

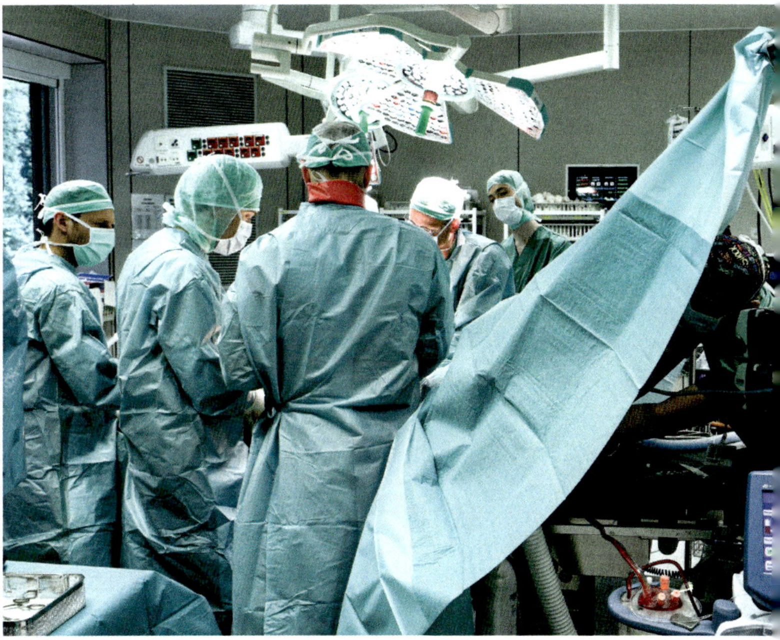

The analogy comes naturally to me. I had the fortune of playing with one of New York's Blues Hall of Famers, Hugh Pool, a prodigious guitarist, vocalist, and bandleader. From him, I learned invaluable lessons about teamwork and leadership. As a bass player, your role is not to stand out, but to make everyone else sound better. You lock in with the drummer, establish the tempo, and hold the groove. When it works, the audience feels the music without quite knowing why. This is exactly how a well-functioning operating room works. Surgeons concentrate fully on anatomy, technique, exposure, and repair. Nurses manage instruments, maintain flow and sterility, and anticipate the next move. Each person plays a crucial role, even if they are not always in the spotlight.

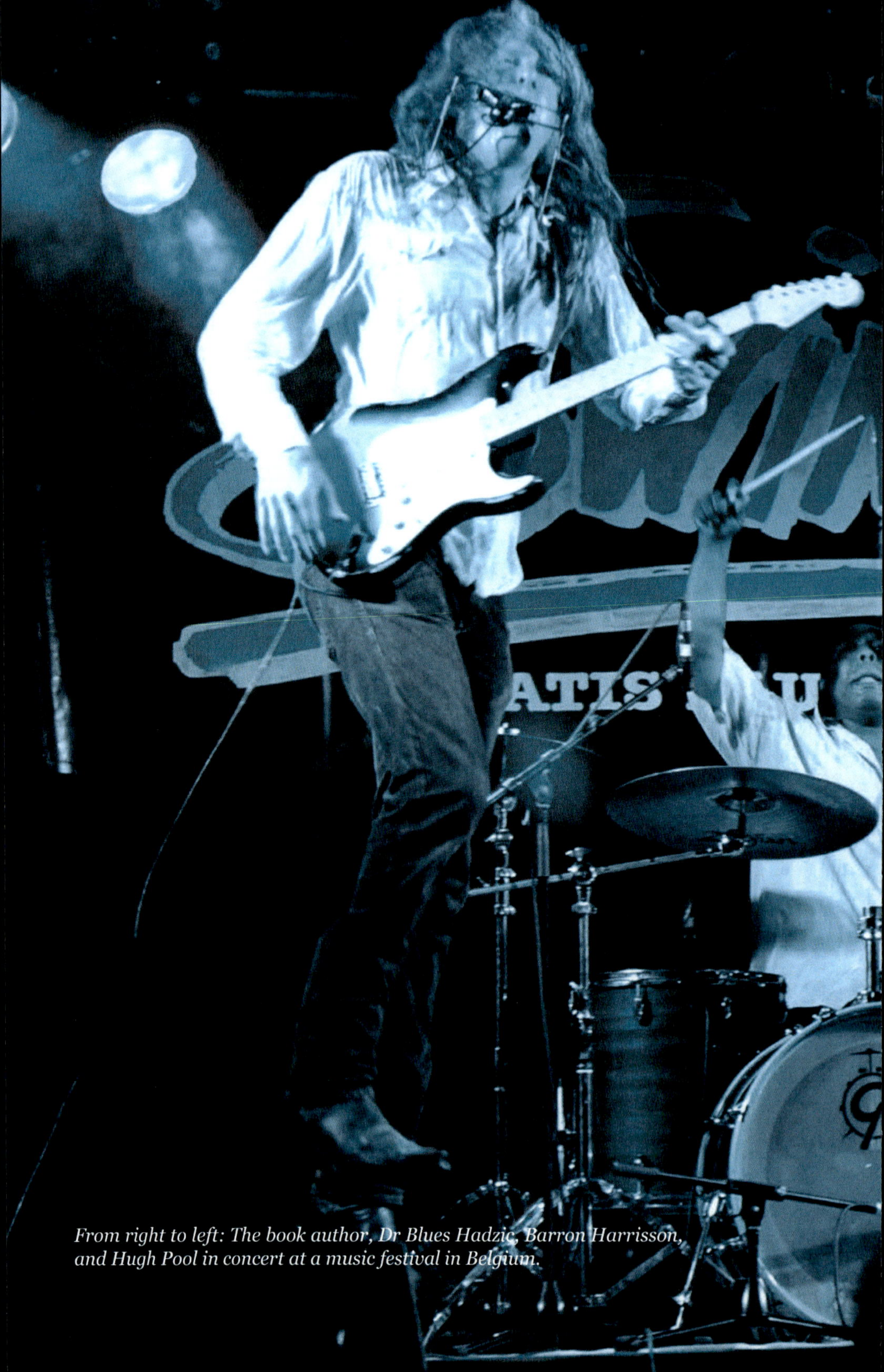

From right to left: The book author, Dr Blues Hadzic, Barron Harrisson, and Hugh Pool in concert at a music festival in Belgium.

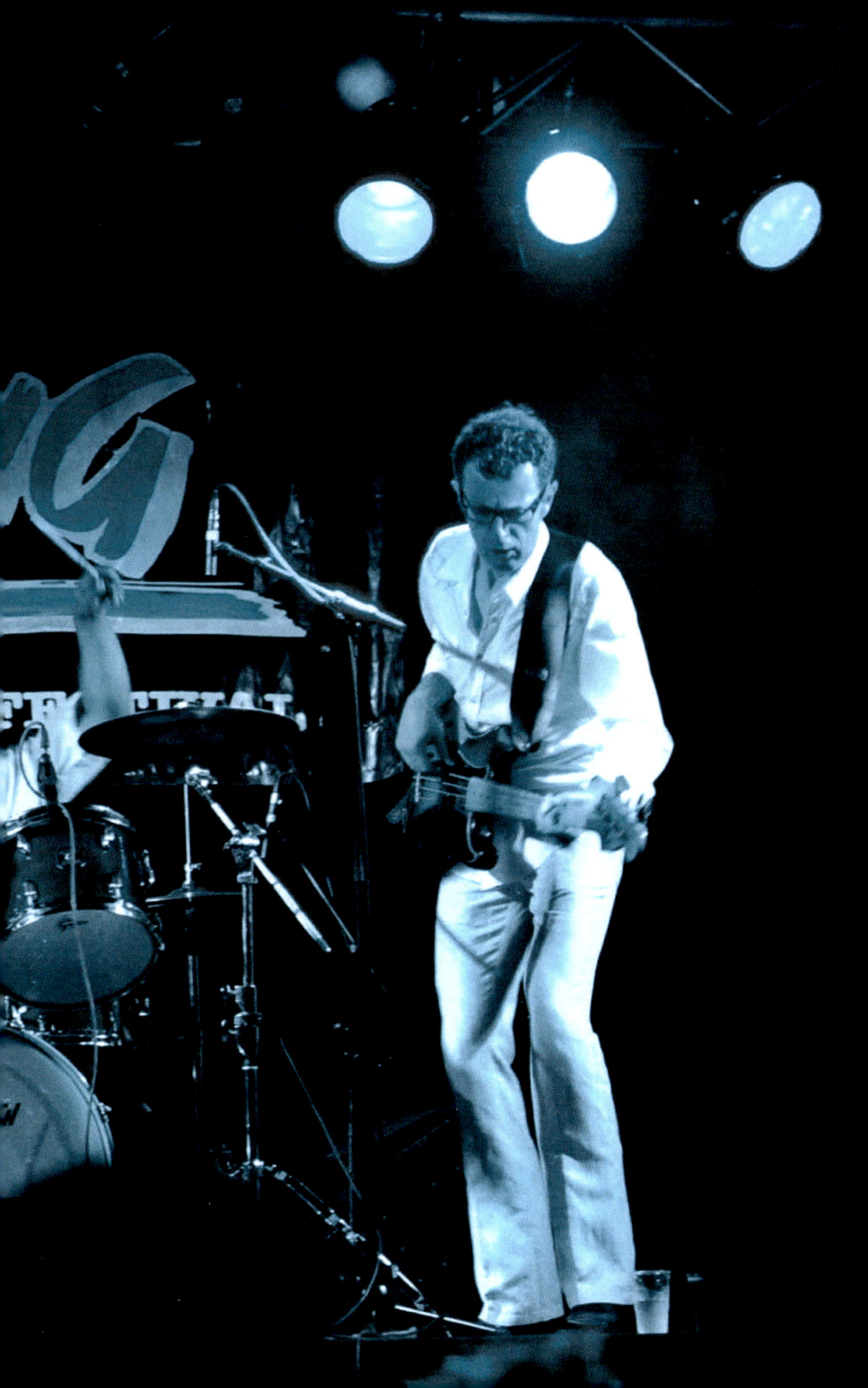

Technicians keep machines alive. Perfusionists stand ready when circulation itself must be taken over.

PACU nurses prepare for the handoff before the case even ends. But at the center of it all, the anesthesiology team sets the tempo.

Anesthesiology is uniquely positioned in the OR ecosystem. We see everything. The patient. The monitors. The surgical field. The blood loss. The pacing of the case. The stress level of the room. We are often the first to sense when rhythm is slipping, when speed outpaces safety, when fatigue creeps in, when communication begins to fray.

A nurse opens a tray before being asked. A tech adjusts a monitor

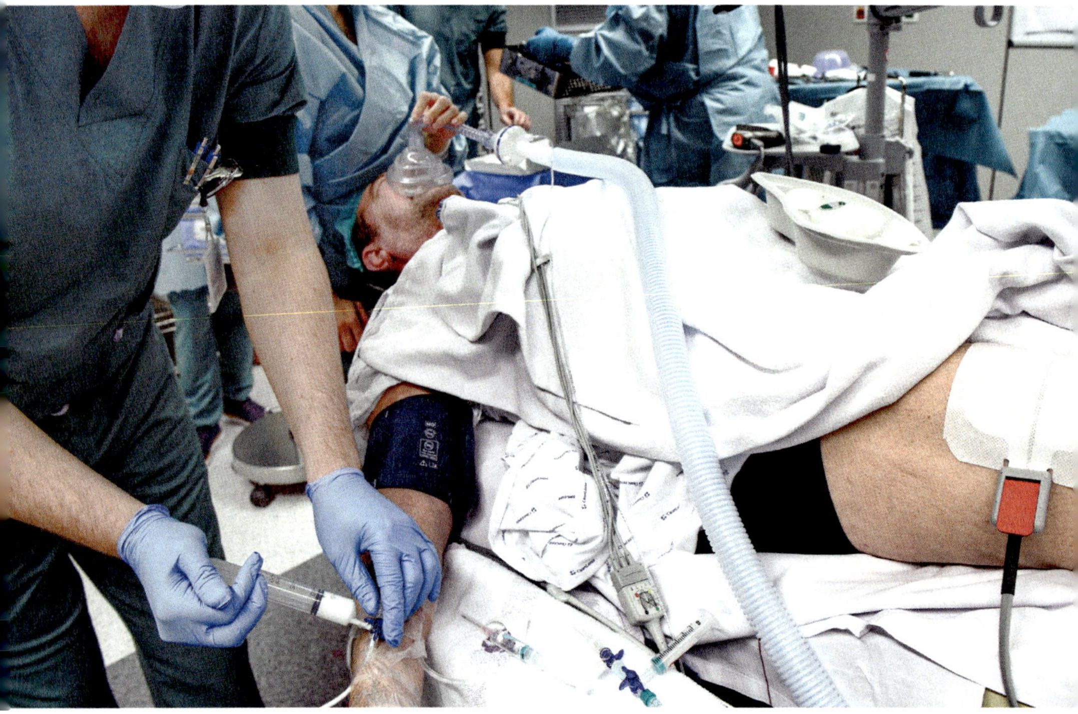

without interrupting. An anesthesia assistant hands equipment before the need is verbalized. A surgeon pauses instinctively when the anesthesiologist says, "Give me a second."

These moments are not accidental. They are the product of trust built over time. And trust in the OR is earned through consistency.

People trust those who behave predictably under pressure. Who do not dramatize. Who communicate clearly and briefly. Leadership in anesthesia is about alignment. Making sure everyone is playing the same song, at the same tempo, for the same patient.

One group deserves special mention here: nurses. If anesthesiologists are the rhythm section, nurses are background vocals.

Operating room does not function without them. They prepare medications meticulously. They position patients with care and dignity. They manage ultrasound equipment, catheters, sterility, documentation, and flow, often simultaneously. They are the silent partners who make nerve blocks anesthesia safe, efficient, and reproducible.

My early mentor and colleague Dr Enio Gallozzi, had little patience for arrogance, but he dealt with it the way only seasoned anesthesiologists do, without raising his voice. When a young surgeon would address him as "Anesthesia," or offer a casual "Good work there, anesthesia," as if approving a background service they scarcely understood, Enio would smile slightly and deliver his line with perfect timing: "A good surgeon deserves a good anesthesiologist. But a bad surgeon, needs one." It landed every time. Not as an insult, but as a correction. In a single sentence, he reminded the room that anesthesiology is not a utility, not a supporting act waiting for praise, but the discipline that holds the line when surgery gets complicated. Most surgeons understood the message immediately and never made the mistake again.

When culture in OR is strong, crises feel contained. When culture is weak, even simple cases feel fragile. Some of the best operating rooms I have worked in were not the newest or best equipped. They were staffed by people who trusted one anoth-

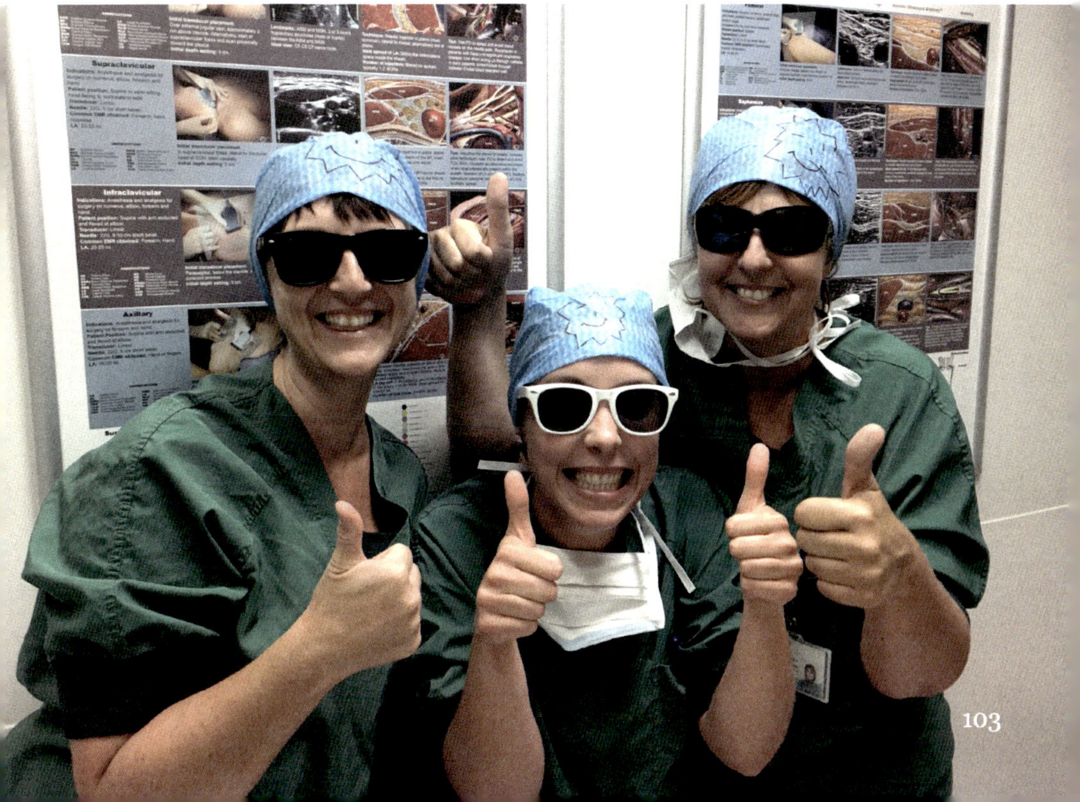

er deeply. People who had learned each other's timing, habits, and tells. People who understood that the goal was not individual excellence, but collective reliability.

Patients sense it. Anxiety drops. Inductions are smoother. Recoveries are easier. Outcomes improve, not because anyone worked harder, but because they worked together.

At the end of the case, when the drapes come down and the patient is transferred to the postoperative care unit (PACU), the rhythm section does not take a bow. The room resets. The next case begins.

Just like music, the magic exists only while it is being played.

Patients remember the soloist. But the surgery only succeeds because the rhythm never stopped.

And that is the job of an anesthesiologist.

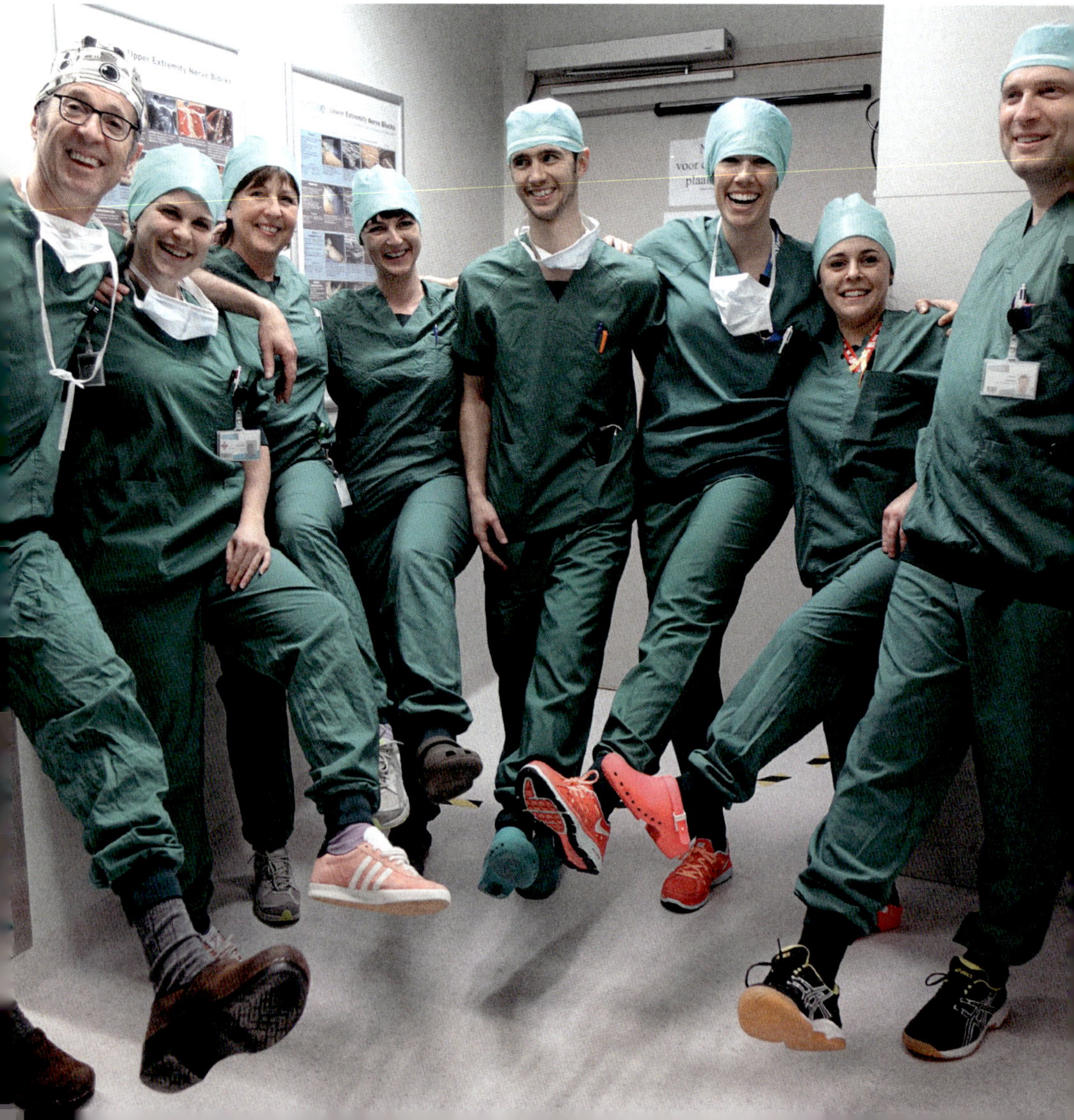

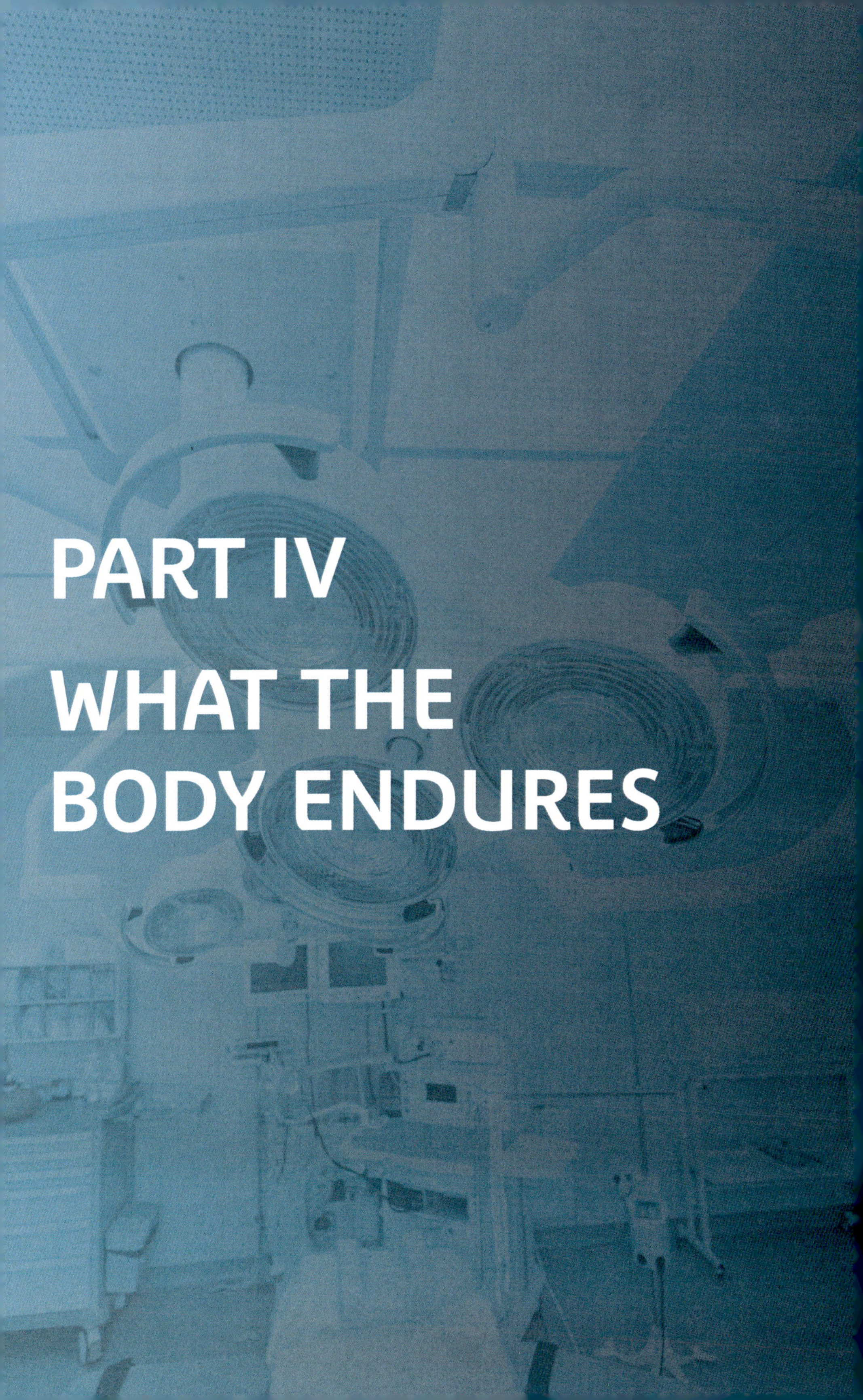

PART IV

WHAT THE BODY ENDURES

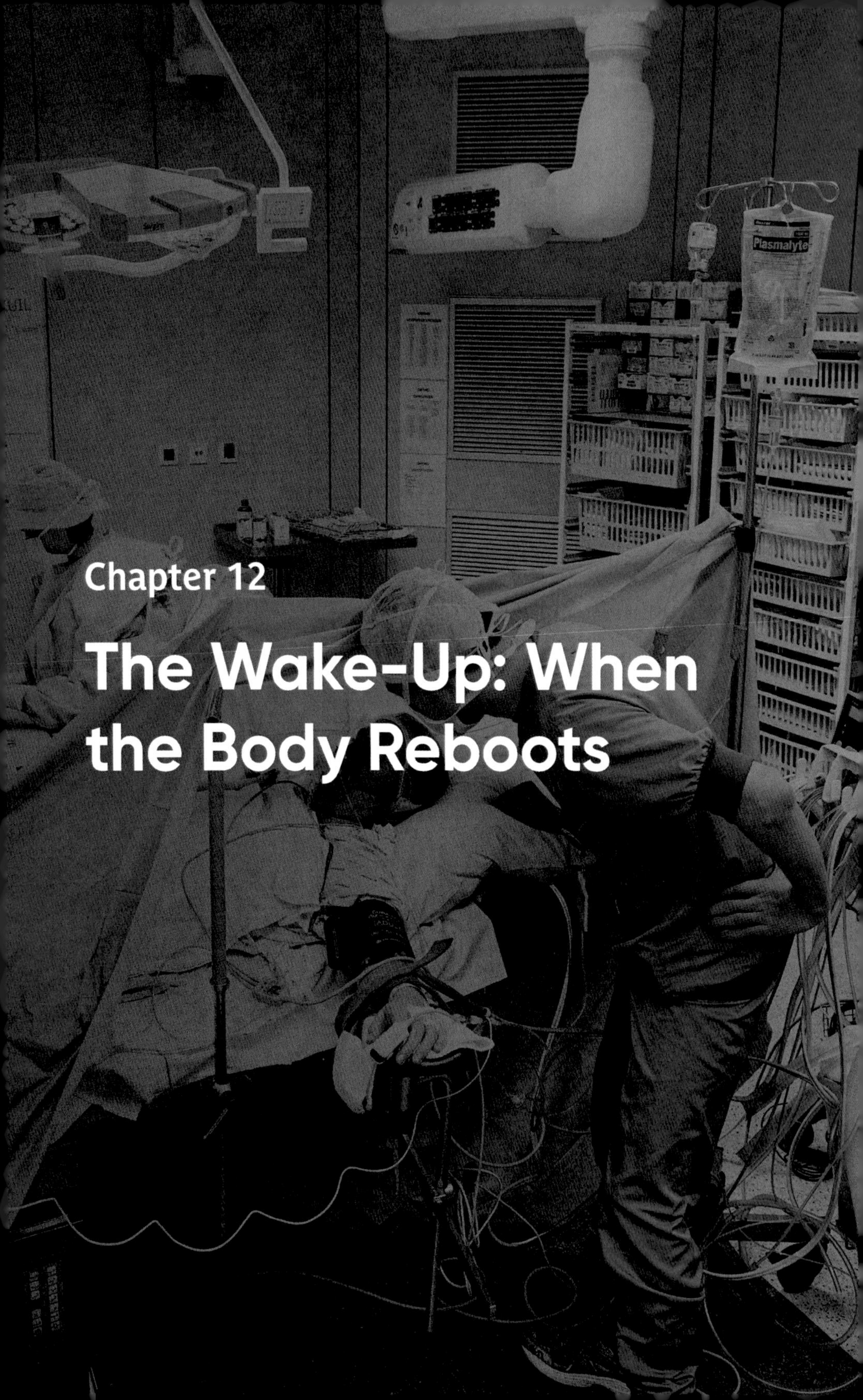

Chapter 12

The Wake-Up: When the Body Reboots

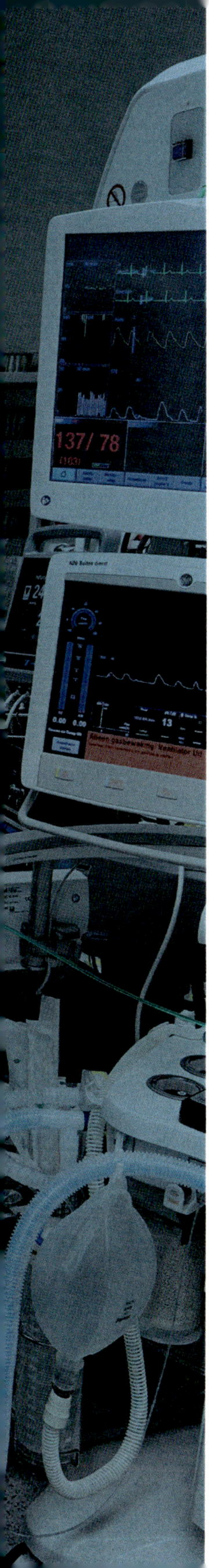

If we buy into the comparison that induction of anesthesia is an airplane take off, and surgery is cruising altitude, then indeed, the wake-up could be considered as landing. And that landing airport is the Post-Anesthesia Care Unit (PACU) is where the body reboots. And the pilots and flight attendants there are PACU nurses.

Recovery does not happen at once. Not predictably. And not always politely or pretty. Faces begin to return - not all at the same speed, not in the same order. Consciousness flickers before it settles. Breathing resumes its own rhythm. The nervous system wakes up and remembers what it does. Immediate post-anesthesia time is a vulnerable moment.

Anesthesia has been lifted, but physiology has not yet fully reassembled itself. Reflexes lag. Airway tone is unreliable. Blood pressure overshoots or undershoots. Pain arrives suddenly, sometimes with urgency. Nausea follows its own logic. The body shivers, not from cold alone, but from thermoregulation finding its reference point again. To the untrained eye, the patient is simply "waking up." To an anesthesiologist and PACU nurse, this is critical, active process.

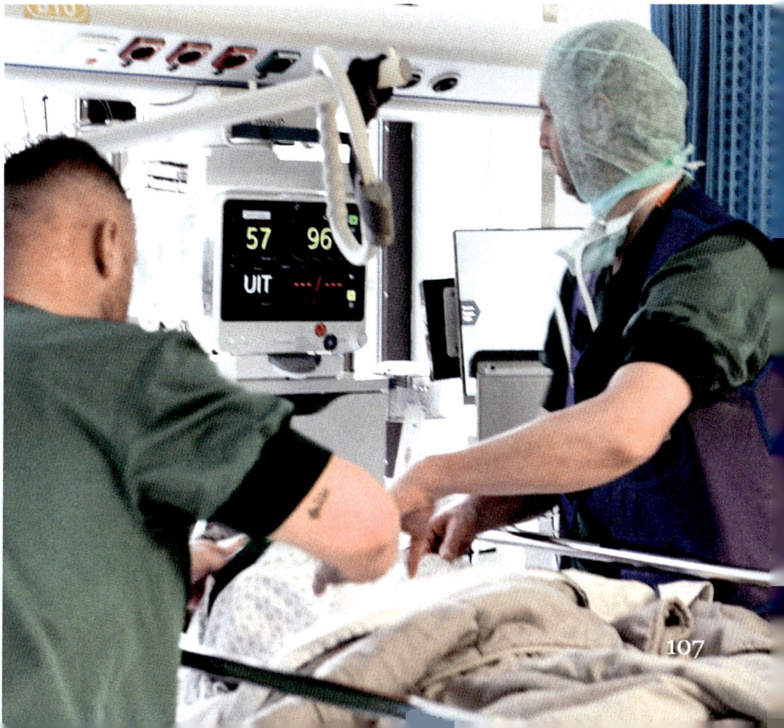

Emergence delirium can look like confusion, agitation, fear, or combativeness. The patient may not recognize where they are or who is speaking to them. Words don't always help. Presence does. A calm voice. Familiar phrases. Reassurance delivered without urgency.

Airway obstruction is common in this phase, and dangerous if missed. A relaxed tongue, residual anesthetic, opioids, sleep apnea revealing itself.

Pain, too, declares itself here. A patient who wakes comfortable moves differently. Breathes differently. Thinks differently. Recovery trajectories diverge early, and PACU and PACU nurses is where that divergence becomes visible.The transfer of the patient from operating room to PACU is not a moment; it is a process. A story passed from one set of hands to another. When

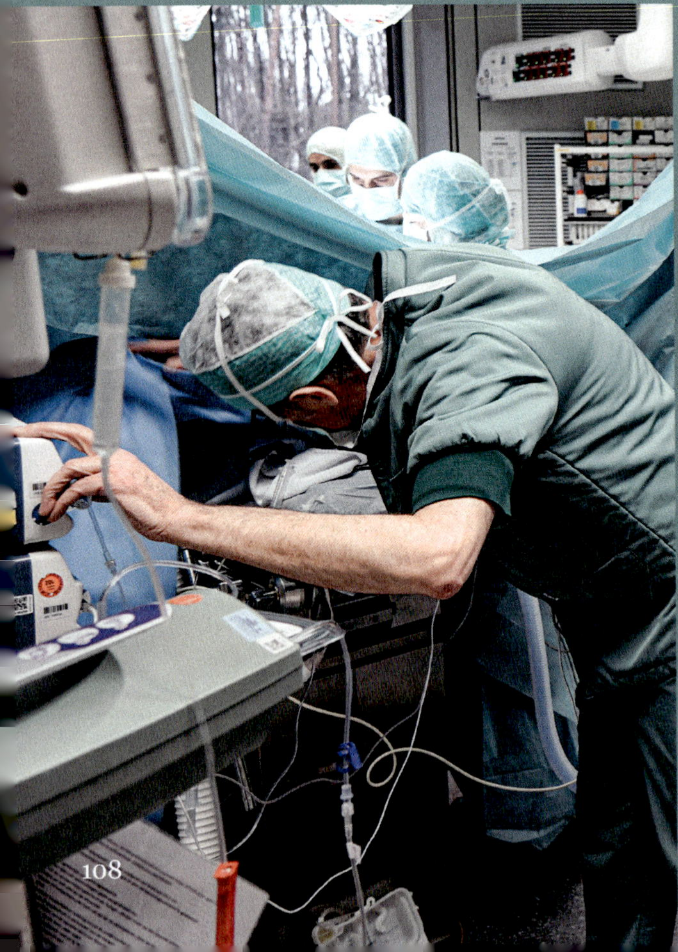

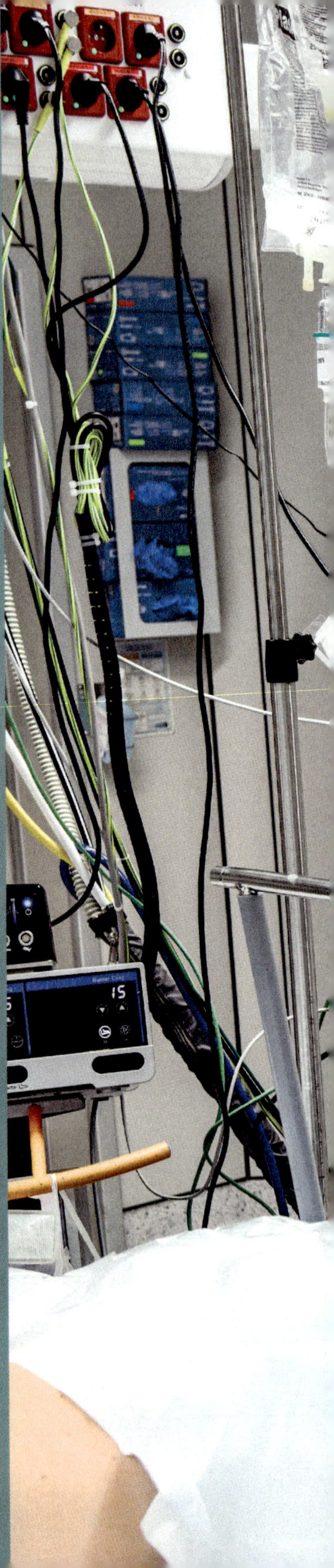

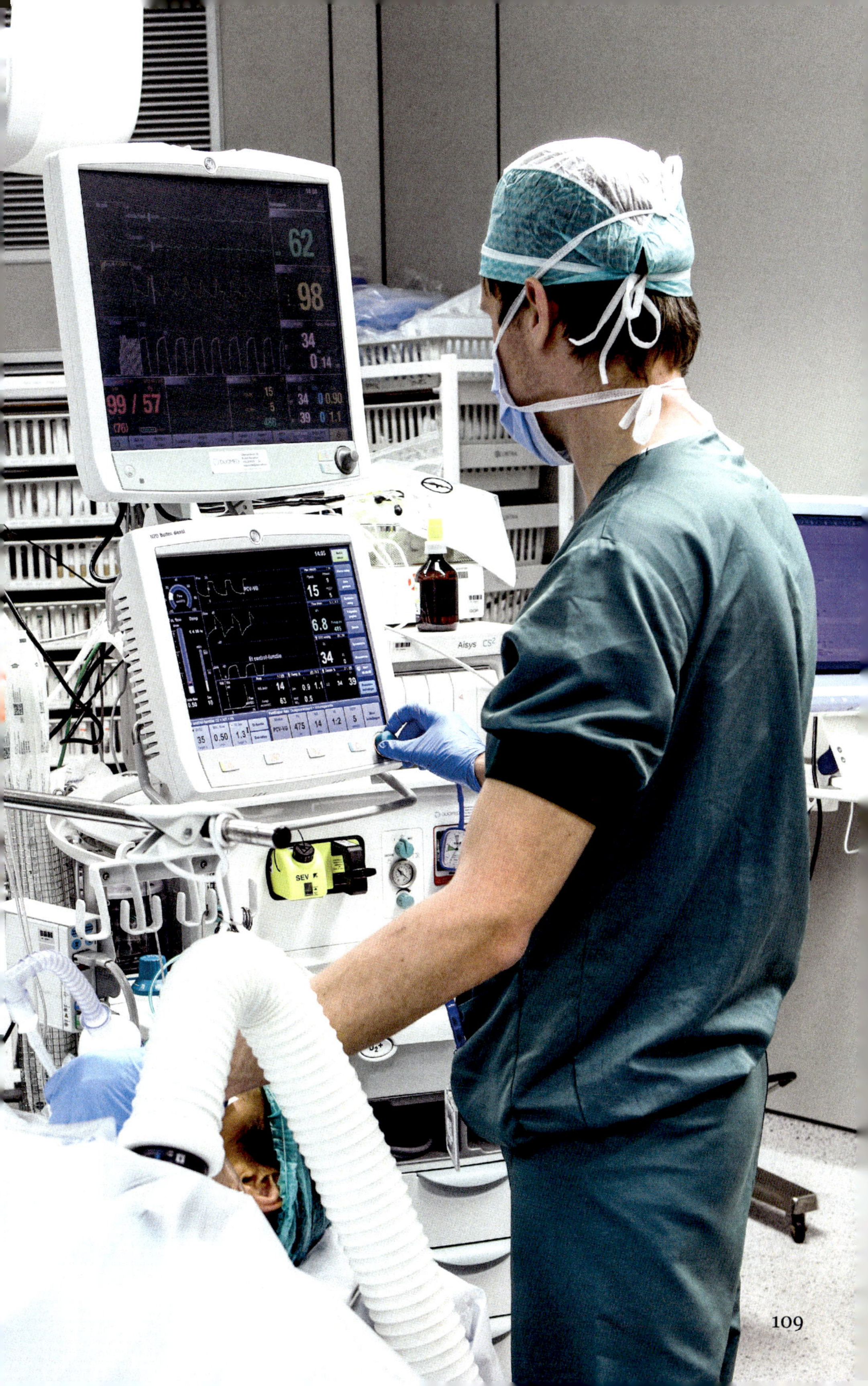
62
98
99 / 57
PCV-VG
Aisys CS²
SEV

done well, it is concise, structured, and respectful. What was done. What matters. What to watch for. What has already been addressed and what has not.

This is where anesthesiology and PACU nurses' culture show itself clearly. PACU nurses are not passive observers; they are expert clinicians who catch what others miss. They see patterns across hundreds of recoveries. They know when something feels off, even before numbers confirm it.

A glance at the airway. A comment about pain trajectory. A quiet mention of something that didn't quite behave as expected. These small exchanges carry disproportionate weight. And PACU nurses are so immensely important in this recovery relationship.

The PACU is the final act of anesthesia. It is where responsibility slowly, but deliberately returns to the patient.

When the anesthesiologist leaves the bedside, it is not abandonment. It is a transfer of trust, executed carefully. The work does not end when the tube comes out or the last anesthetic is turned off. It ends when the patient is stable, and protected by a team ready to take over.

Eventually, the monitors quiet down again. Curtains open. Family members appear. The patient speaks. Remembers. Complains. Laughs. Asks for water.

Life resumes.

And like so much in anesthesiology, if the wake-up goes well, it looks like nothing special happened at all.

That, quietly, is the success of the landing.

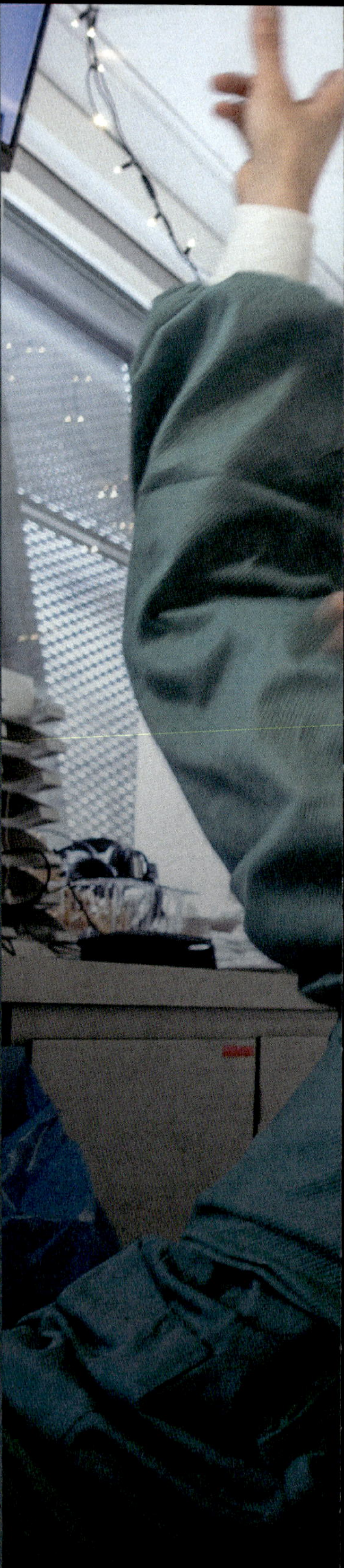

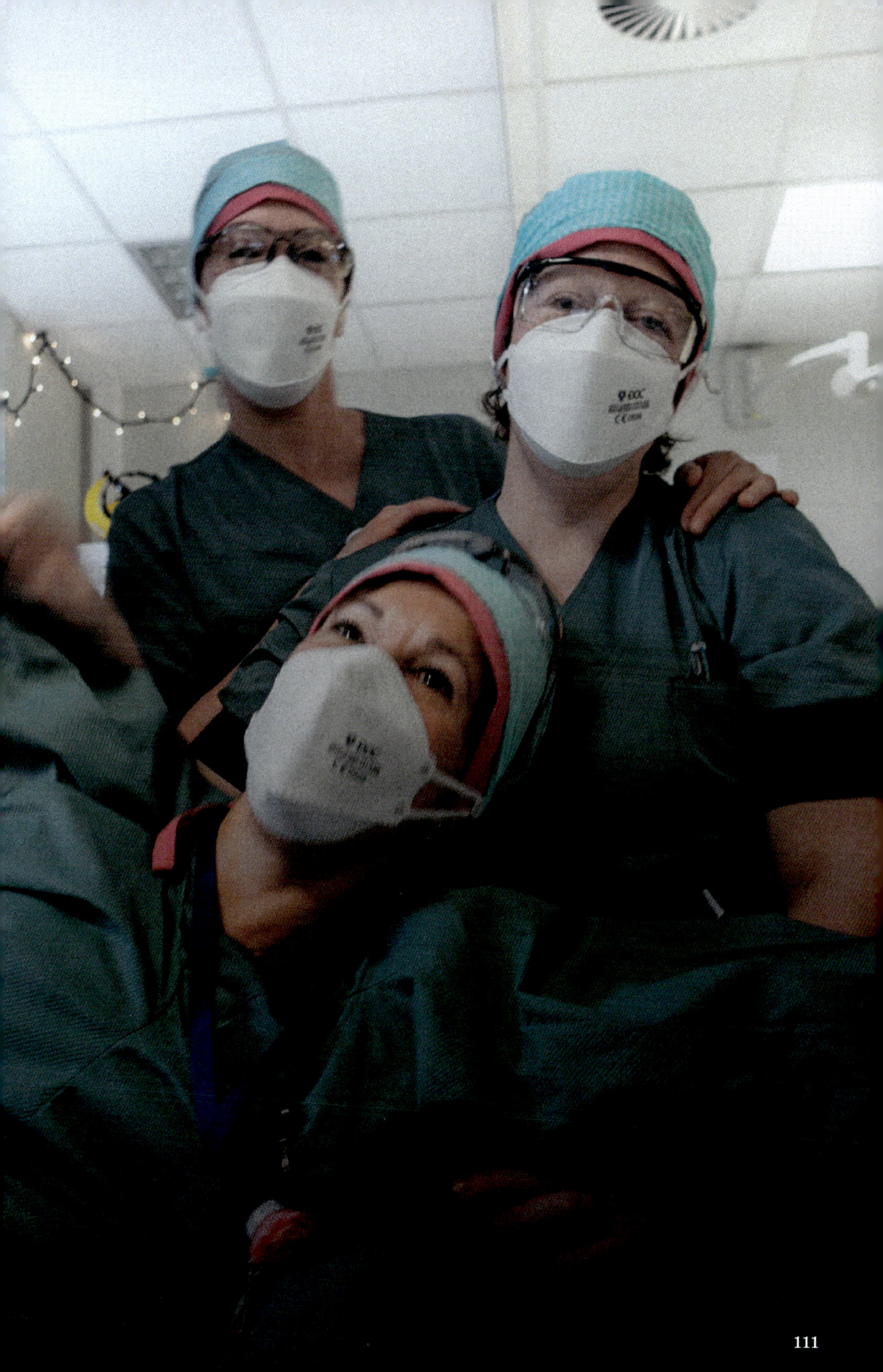

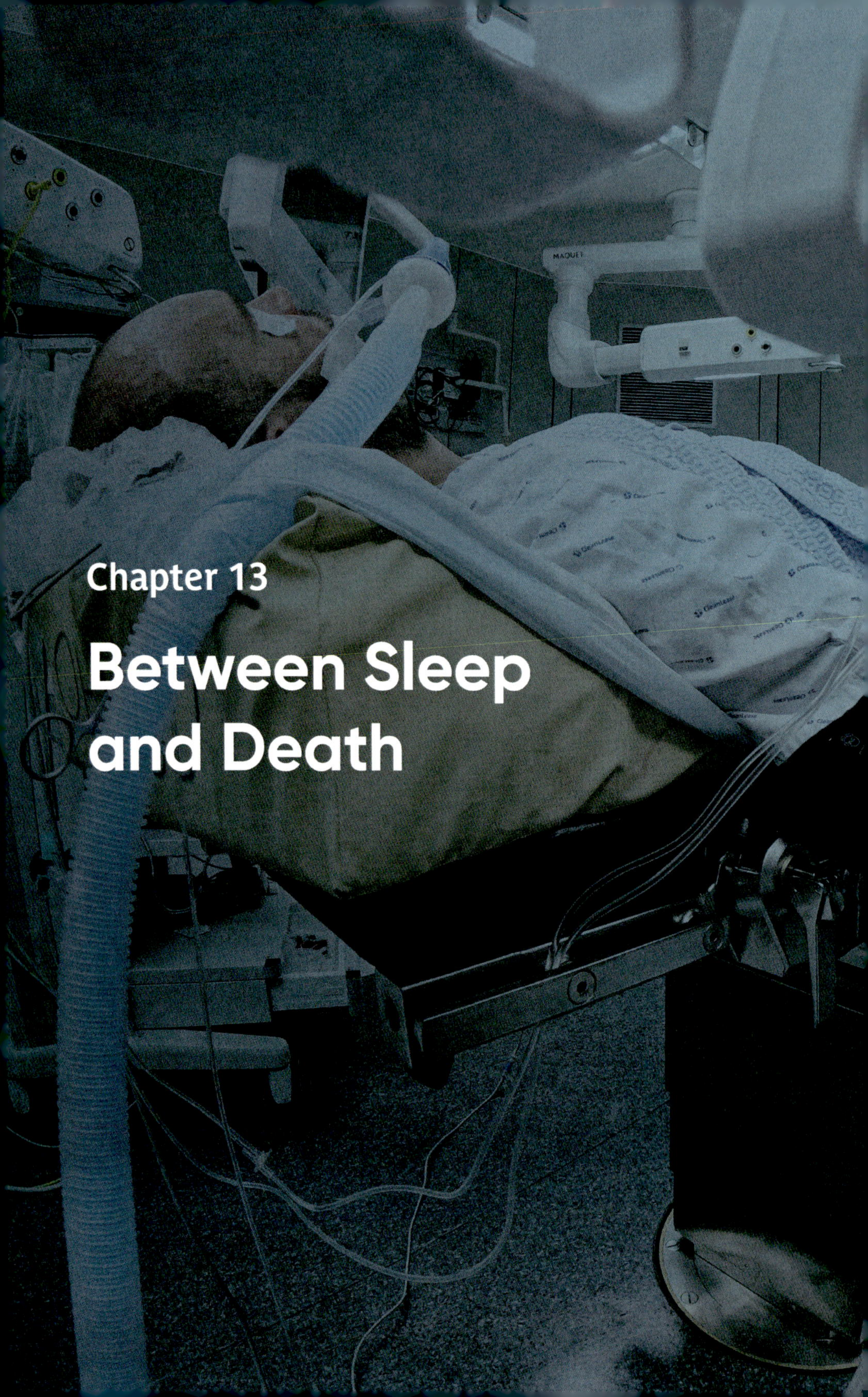

Chapter 13

Between Sleep and Death

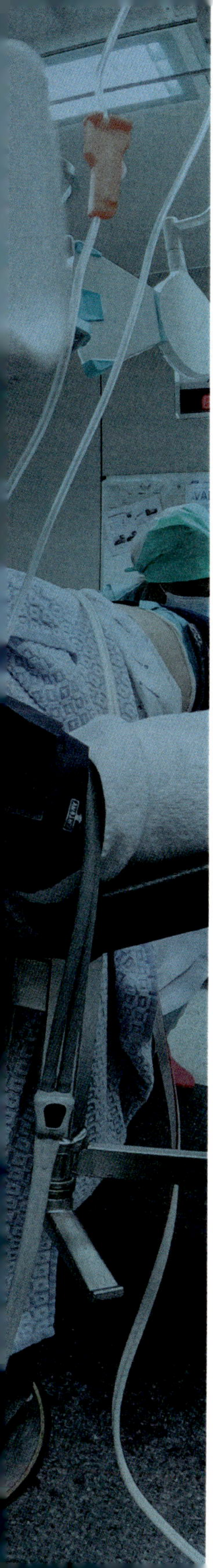

Most people think anesthesia is a kind of sleep.

It isn't. Sleep is something the body knows how to do on its own. You lie down, close your eyes, and consciousness fades while breathing, blood pressure, reflexes, and temperature quietly take care of themselves. Anesthesia is different. Under anesthesia, those natural protections are deliberately weakened or temporarily taken over entirely.

That is why anesthesia is both life-saving and inherently dangerous. Under general anesthesia, consciousness is not simply turned off. The brain is placed into an altered state where awareness, pain perception, and memory are suppressed. But the price of that suppression is profound: the same medications that block pain and consciousness also interfere with breathing, circulation, temperature control, muscle strength, and protective reflexes that keep a person alive.

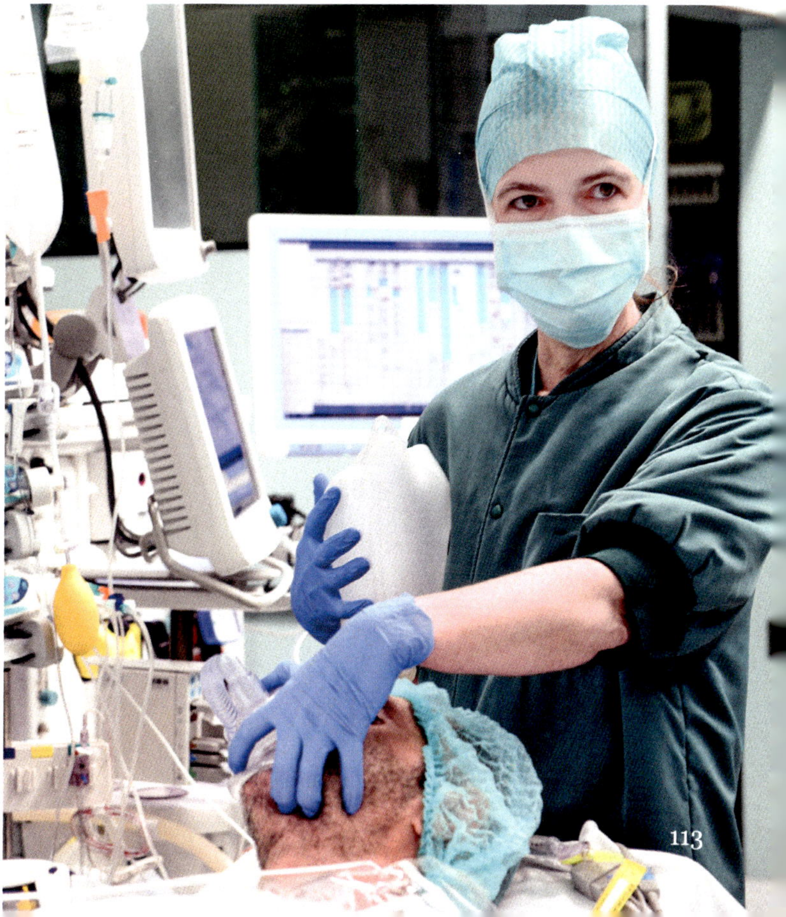

Most anesthetic medications and gasses reduce or abolish the drive to breathe. The chest no longer rises reliably on its own. The normal amount of CO_2 and oxygen that we breath in and out decreases to dangerous levels, at which a person would not survive without an intervention. Airway muscles relax. The tongue falls back, further preventing or stopping the breathing. Coughing and swallowing, reflexes that normally protect the lungs, fade and then completely disappear. Left alone, an anesthetized person would quickly suffocate and die due to hypoxia, hypocarbia, hypothermia, and circulation arrest.

There is an uncomfortable truth about anesthesia that is rarely stated plainly. The same medications used to produce anesthesia in carefully measured doses, are closely related to those used in death sentence executions by lethal injection. The difference is typically not the medications; the difference is intervention.

So the anesthesiologist takes over.

A breathing tube or mask is utilized to deliver oxygen. A breathing machine takes over the rhythm of respiration. Every breath becomes intentional, measured, adjusted moment by moment based on what

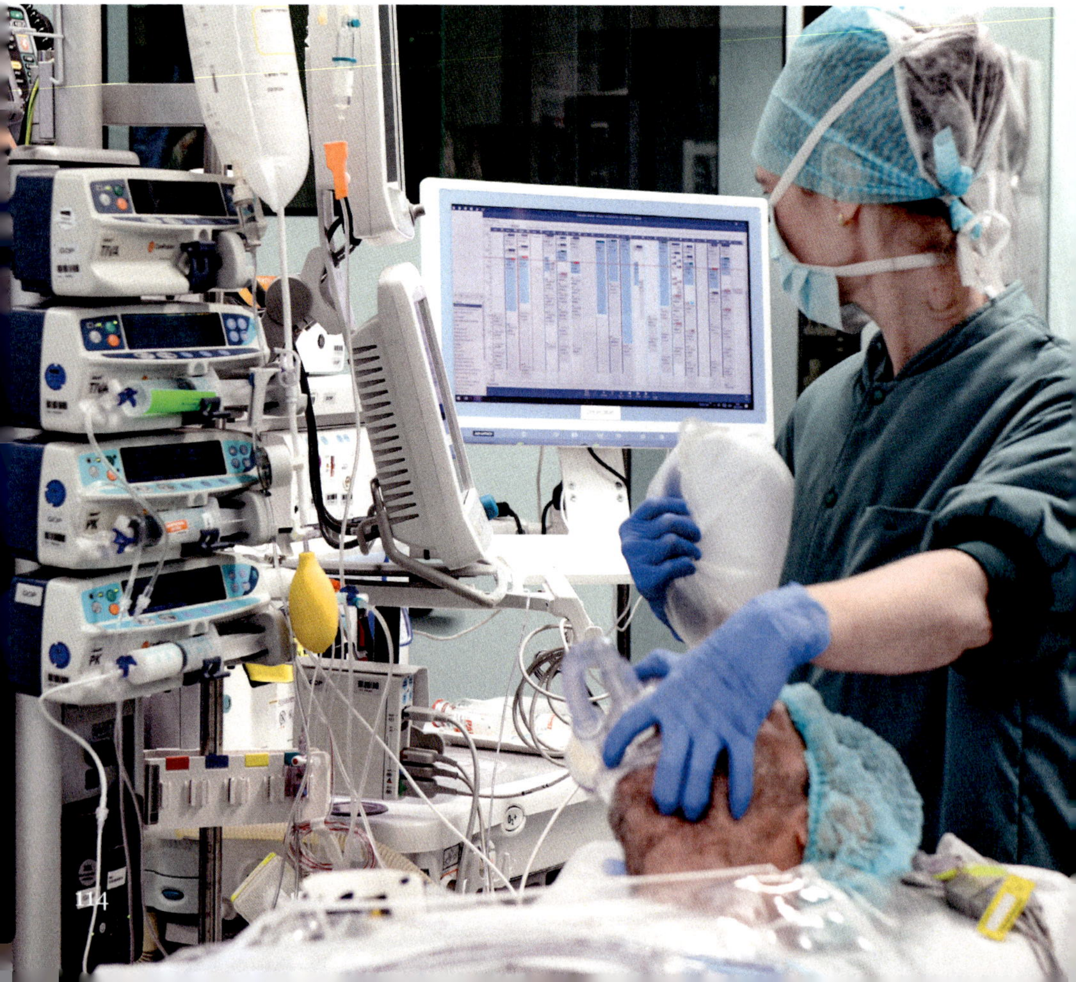

the body shows in return on sophisticated respiratory and cardiovascular monitors. Oxygen in. Carbon dioxide out. Not too much. Not too little.

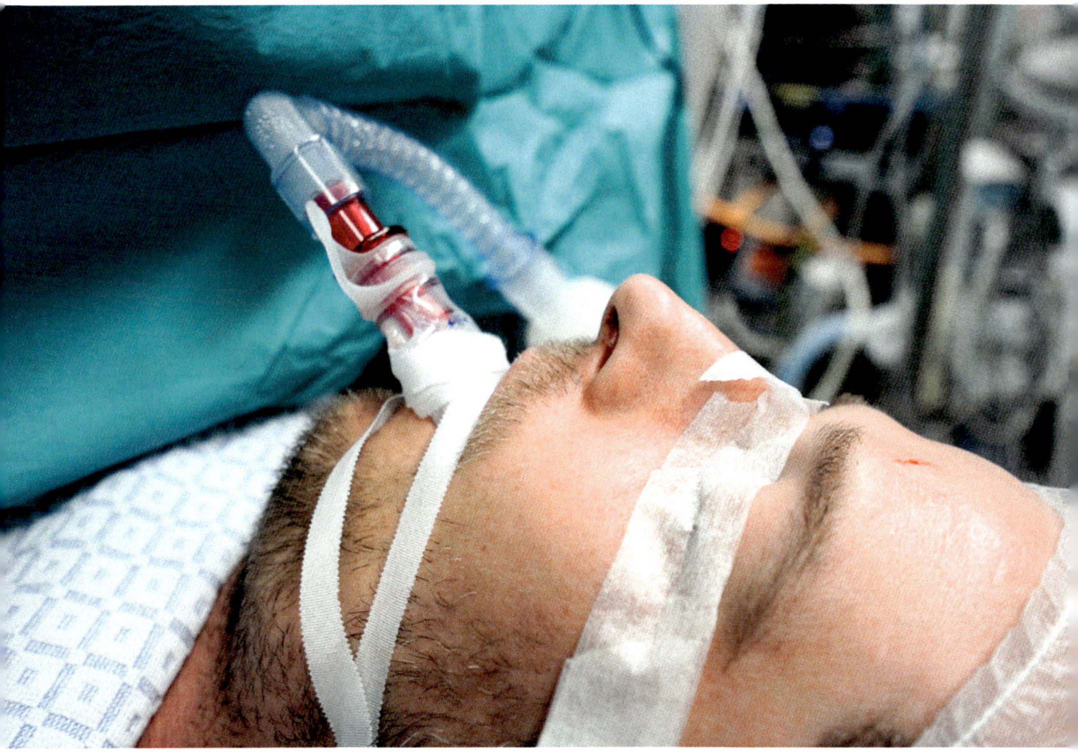

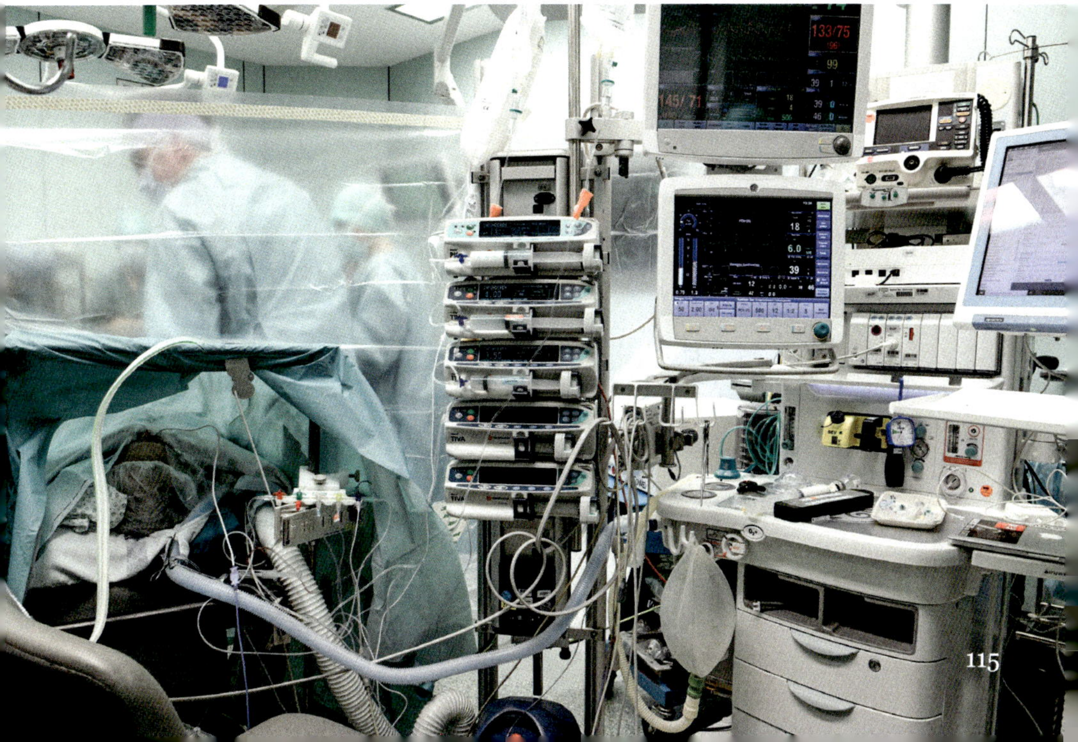

Most anesthetic medications lower blood pressure by relaxing blood vessels and weakening the heart's pumping strength. It is intrinsic to how these agents work. In healthy patients undergoing anesthesia and surgery, the body somewhat compensates to a certain degree. In others, the cardiac physiology fails quickly. That is why anesthesiology professionals watch blood pressure constantly. Fluids, medications, and adjustments are made continuously to maintain blood flow to organs that cannot tolerate even short interruption of blood and oxygen delivery - brain, heart, kidneys...

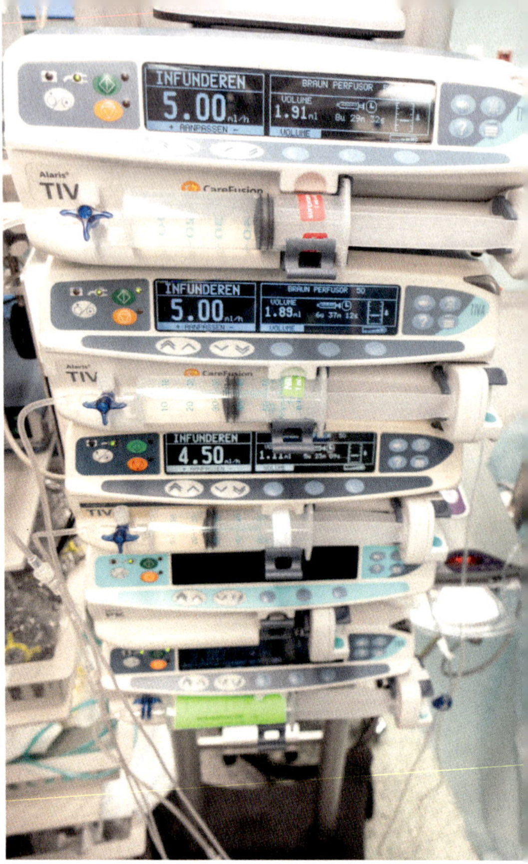

Temperature is another silent casualty.

When you are cold, your body shivers reflectively to increase the metabolism, produce heat and keep the tem-

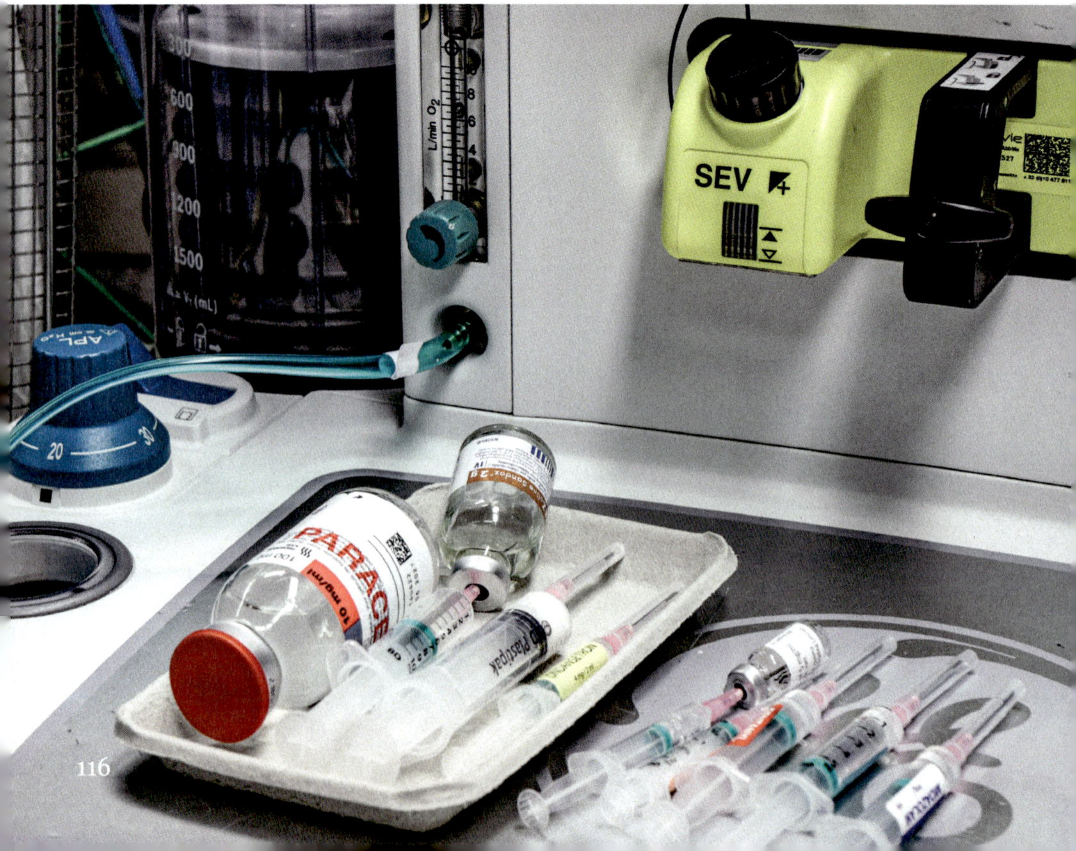

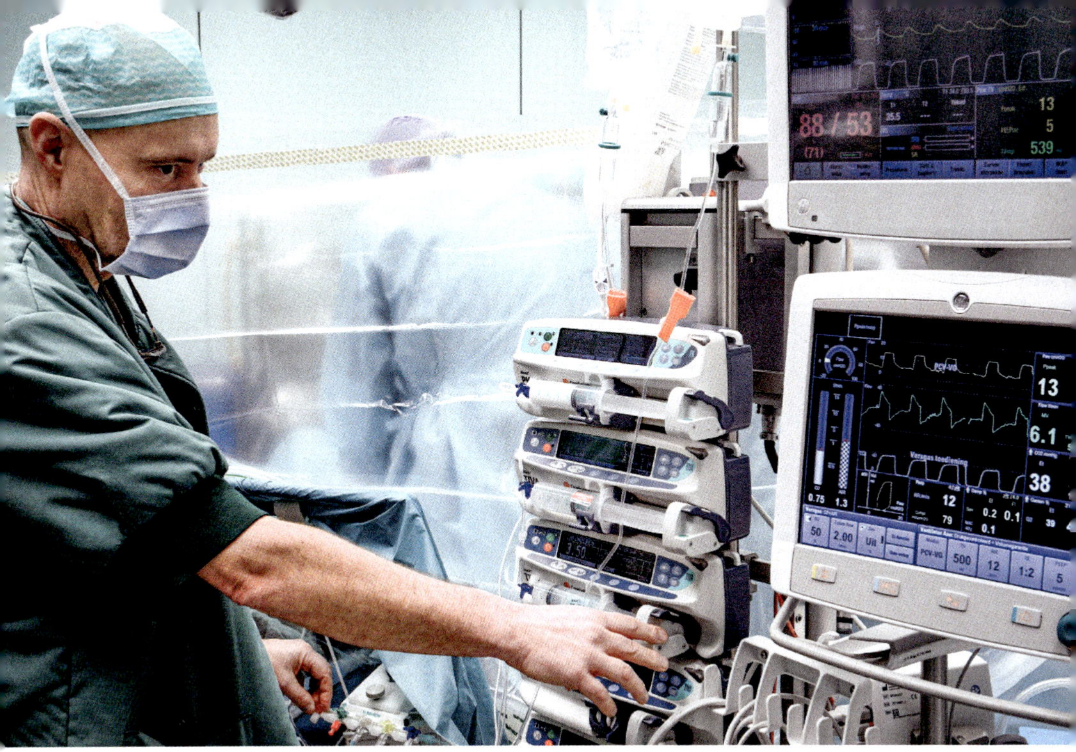

perature stable. Under anesthesia, the body loses its ability to regulate heat. Blood vessels dilate. Heat escapes. Shivering mechanisms are disabled and a patient can become dangerously cold without feeling it or ability to self-correct it. That is why warming blankets, fluid warmers, forced air warming, and temperature monitoring probes are always used during anesthesia and operation; not for comfort, but for survival.

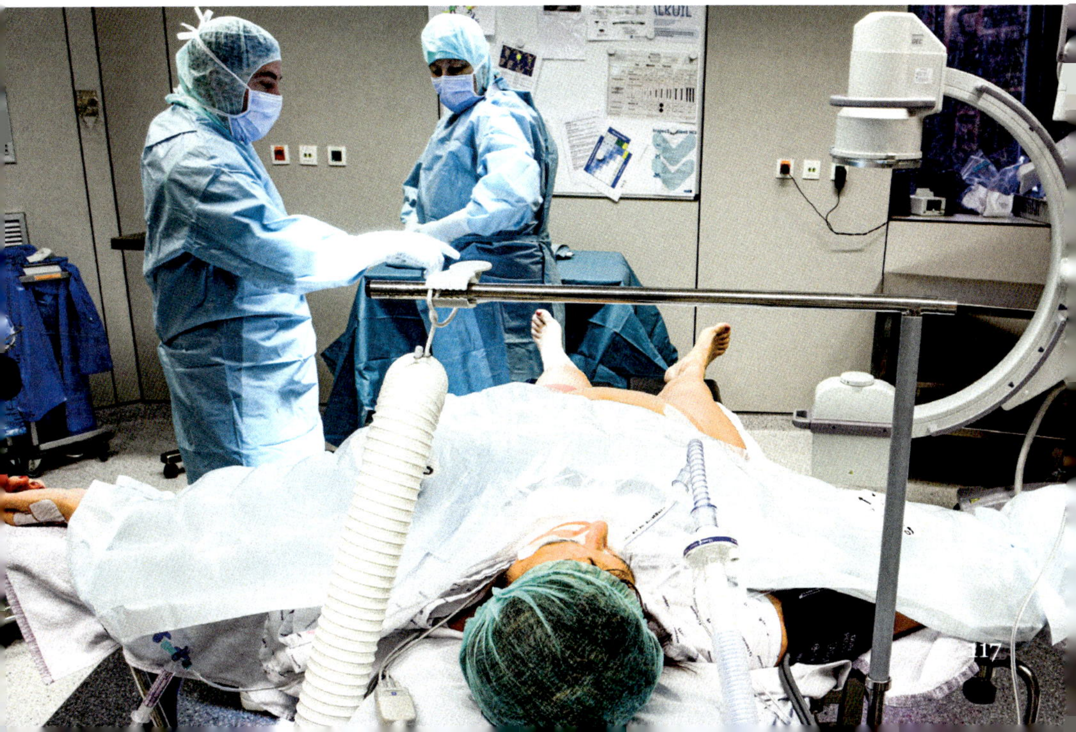

Natural, protected reflexes disappear as well.

The blink reflex. The gag reflex. The response to pain. These are not inconveniences, they are safeguards to an awake individual. Administration of anesthesia temporarily suspends them to allow surgery, then carefully restores them in reverse order at the end of the operation. Too much suppression, too long, and the consequences are serious. Too little, and suffering or awareness becomes possible.

This balance is what makes anesthesia a craft rather than a switch. But get this: There is no single depth or dose of anesthesia that fits every patient or every moment. Surgical stimulation changes. Blood loss changes. Position changes. The anesthesiologist adjusts the physiology continuously, often before your body signals distress in obvious ways, when the reversal becomes much more challenging and/or dangerous.

An anesthetic is not something you "give" and walk away from. This is why the code of anesthetic practice mandates the anesthesiologist to be present throughout the entire conductance of an anesthetic. Every anesthetic is a live experiment unfolding in real time, guided by training, experience, and constant observation.

Without an anesthesiologist, anesthesia would be lethal. With one, it becomes transformative.

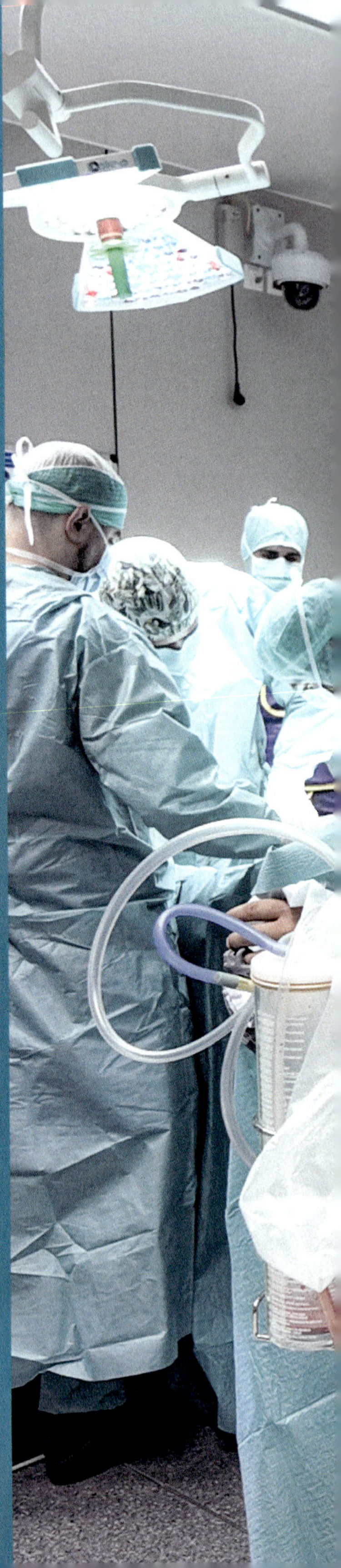

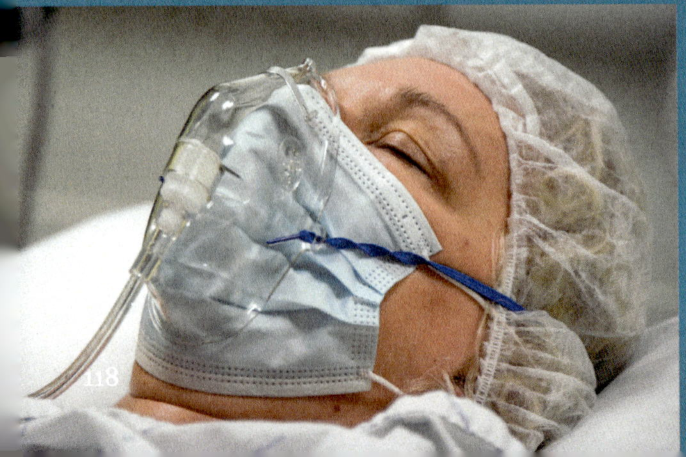

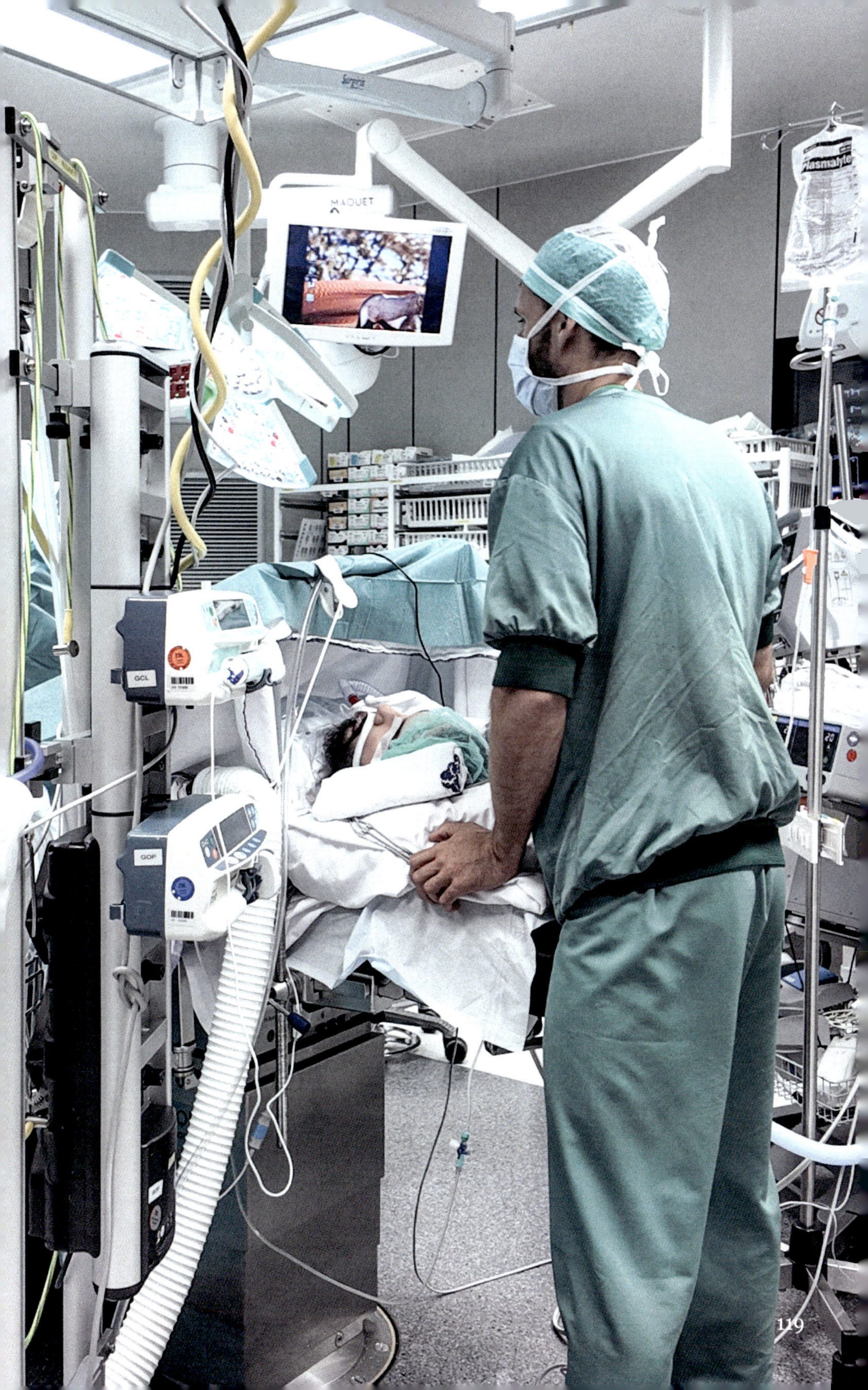

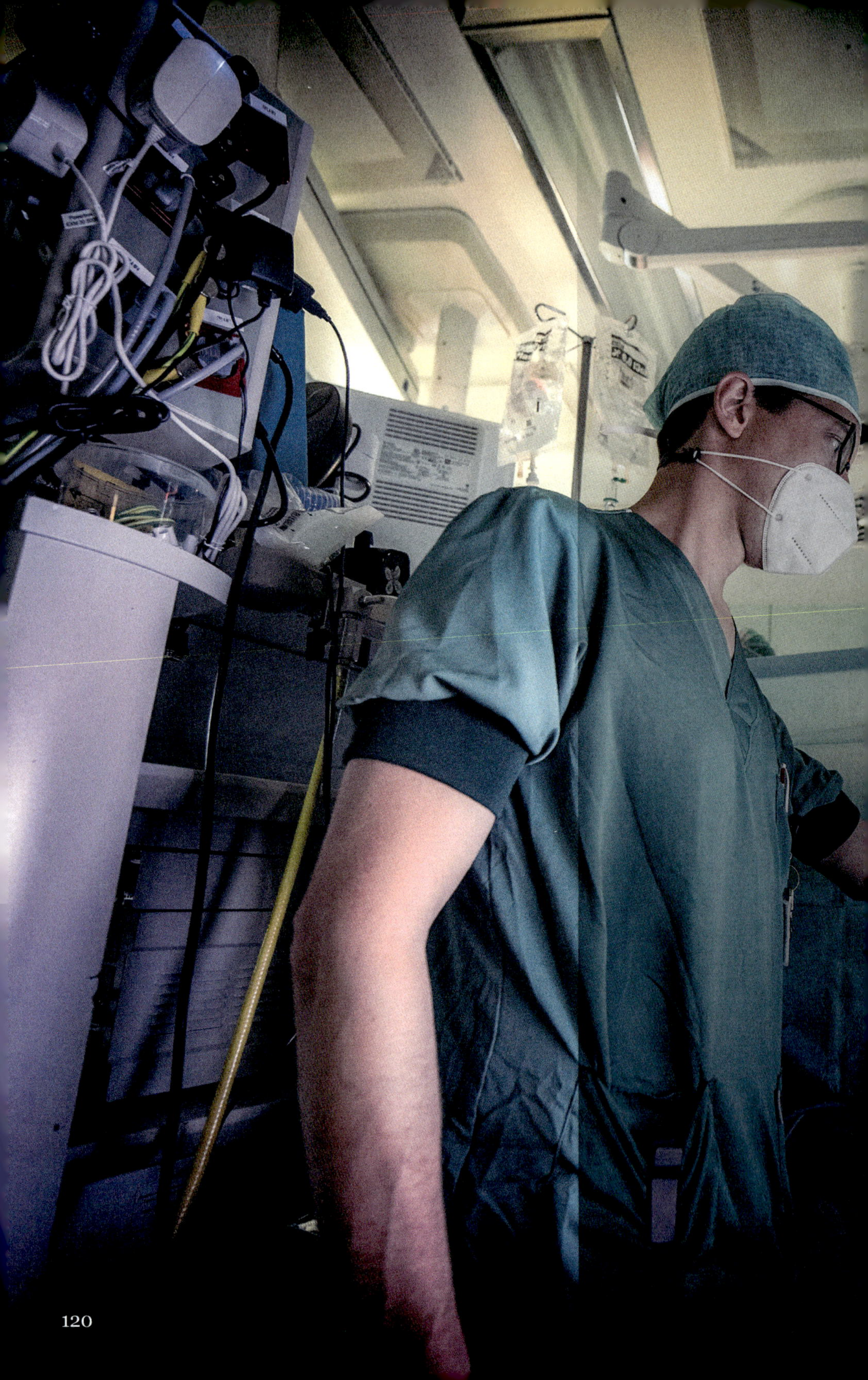

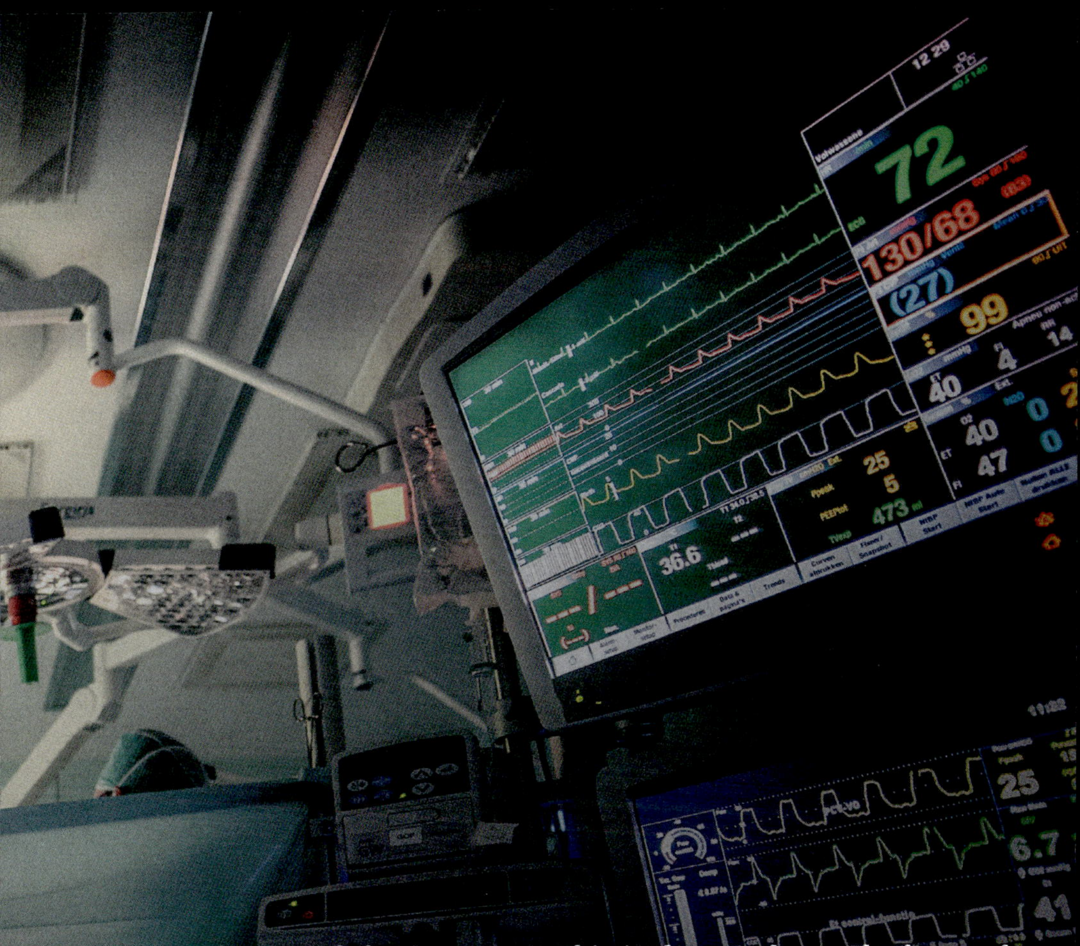

To get a glimpse of the immense responsibility that anesthesiology practitioners exercise daily, try to imagine yourself in an environment such as the one pictured, where every decision you make and every button you press has an effect on another human being. A person who has put his or her life into your hands and who is now 100% dependent on the decisions YOU make.

Anesthesia allows patients to pass through procedures their bodies could not otherwise tolerate. It makes modern medicine possible, but only because someone is continuously protecting the systems anesthesia deliberately disrupts.

This is the paradox at the heart of anesthesiology. When patients wake up, they often say, "It felt like I just fell asleep." But, behind this oversimplification, it lies a complex, fragile balance, maintained, continuously, and deliberately by someone who is trained to make sure the body survives a state it was never meant to endure on its own.

That is what anesthesia really is.

Not sleep.

But controlled vulnerability, watched over until the body can safely take itself back.

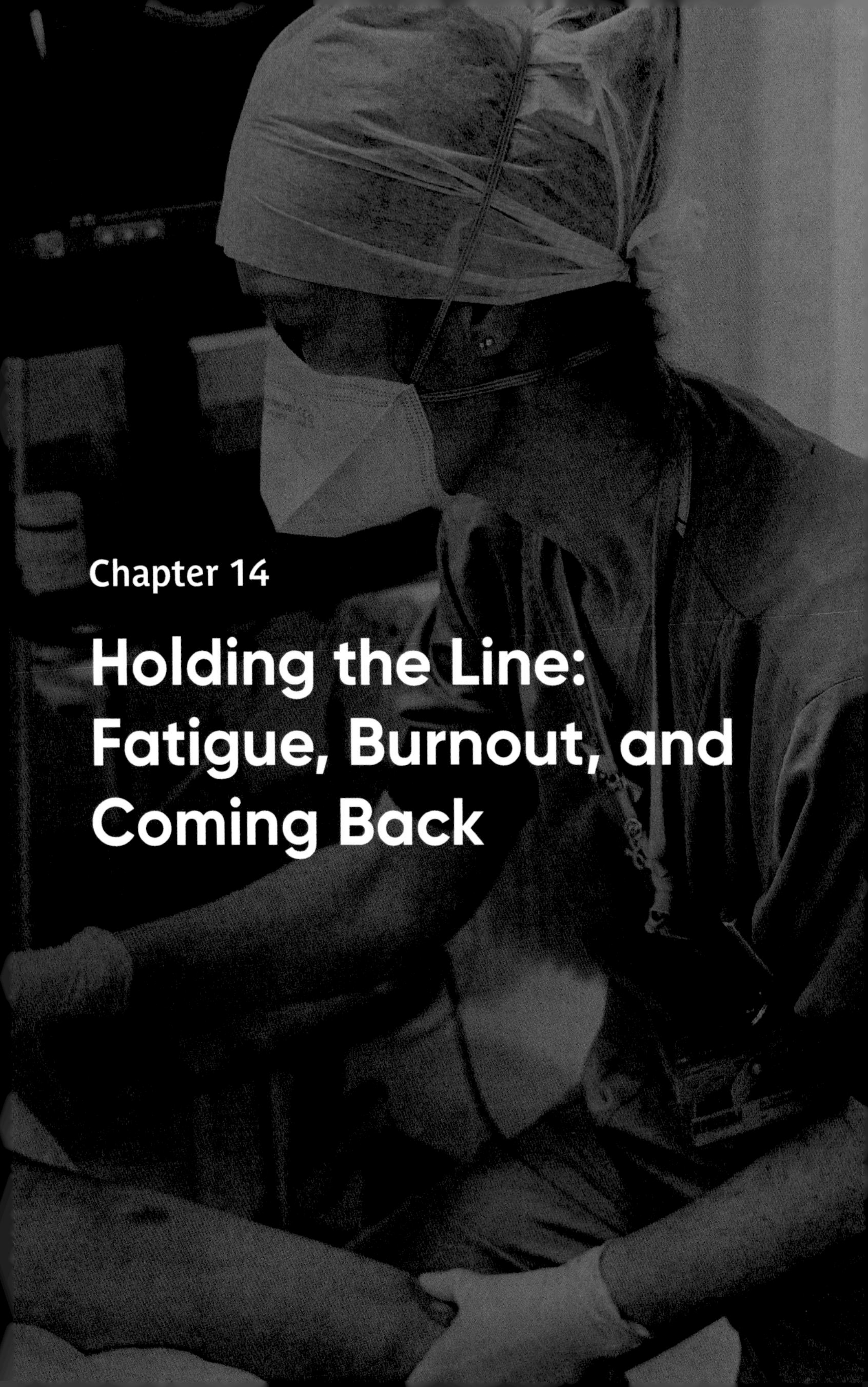

Chapter 14

Holding the Line: Fatigue, Burnout, and Coming Back

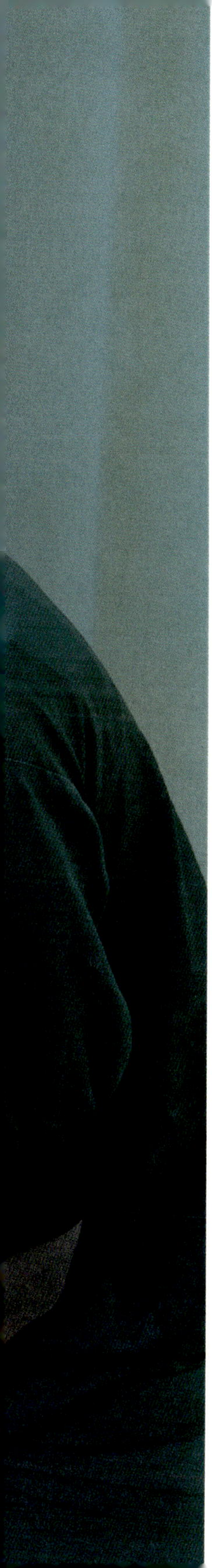

Practicing anesthesiology is physical, and yet, it does not exhaust your body first.

It exhausts the mind.

The physical demands are obvious; long hours, night call, standing still for extended periods, moving equipment, moving and positioning patients, responding instantly when things change. But the deeper fatigue comes from something less visible: sustained act of watching, anticipating, and decision-making, without much pause.

Night call makes this reality unmistakable.

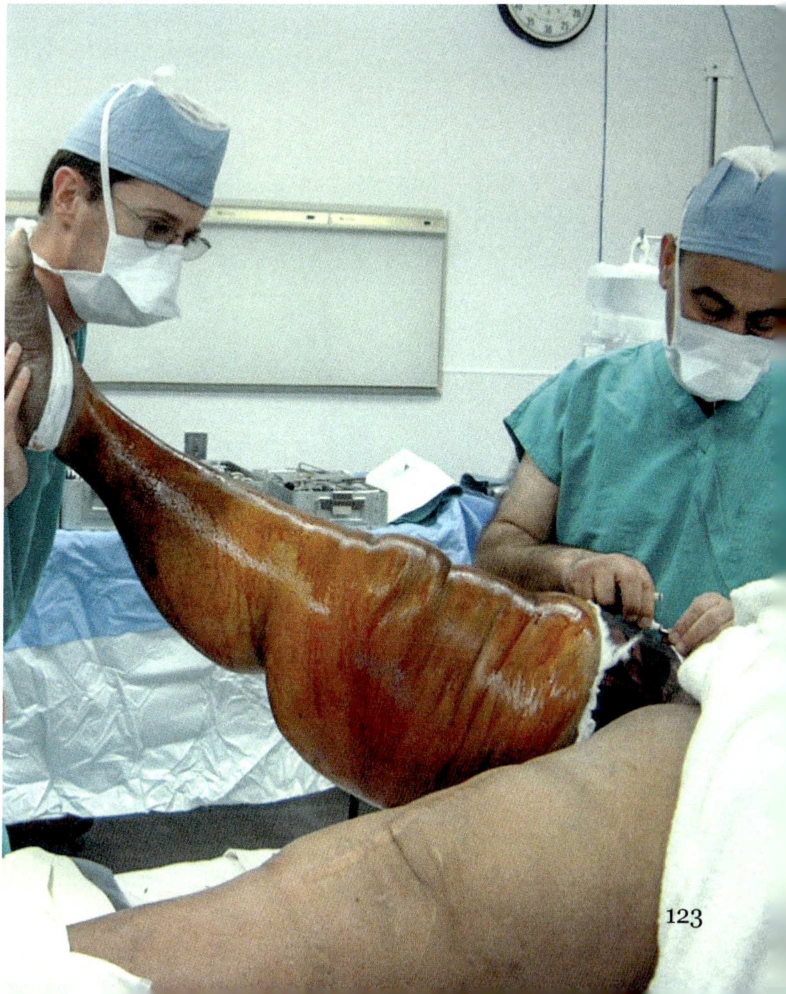

Hospitals at night feel different. Corridors stretch longer. Voices drop. Time loses its usual structure. You move from bright operating rooms to dim ICUs, from urgent phone calls to long, silent stretches interrupted by sudden intensity. Sleep, when it comes, is often shallow and provisional, never complete. As the next page or phone call carries another challenge, emergency that must be dealt with timely. Even for the very experienced anesthesiologists, with years of clinical practice behind their belt, every phone call carries a dose of stress of the unknown set of interventions and decisions that await seconds or minutes right after that call.

And yet, the standard of care is always the same. Day or night. Rested or exhausted. Whether it's the first case of the morning or the last emergency before dawn, the expectations are exactly the same. There is no allowance for fatigue, no adjustment for lost sleep. The physiology doesn't care, and neither does the responsibility.

That is what night duty makes unmistakably clear.

At midnight, physiology does not become more forgiving. Decisions do not slow down. The expectation is unchanged: clarity, calm and precision. This is where cognitive load accumulates.

Anesthesiologists juggle dozens of variables at once: ventilation, circulation, medications, surgical progress, patient positioning, comorbidities, what has already occurred, and constant anticipation of what is likely to happen next. The mental simulations running constantly in the background often go unseen and unchecked. Constant corrections of physiology derailment that must be

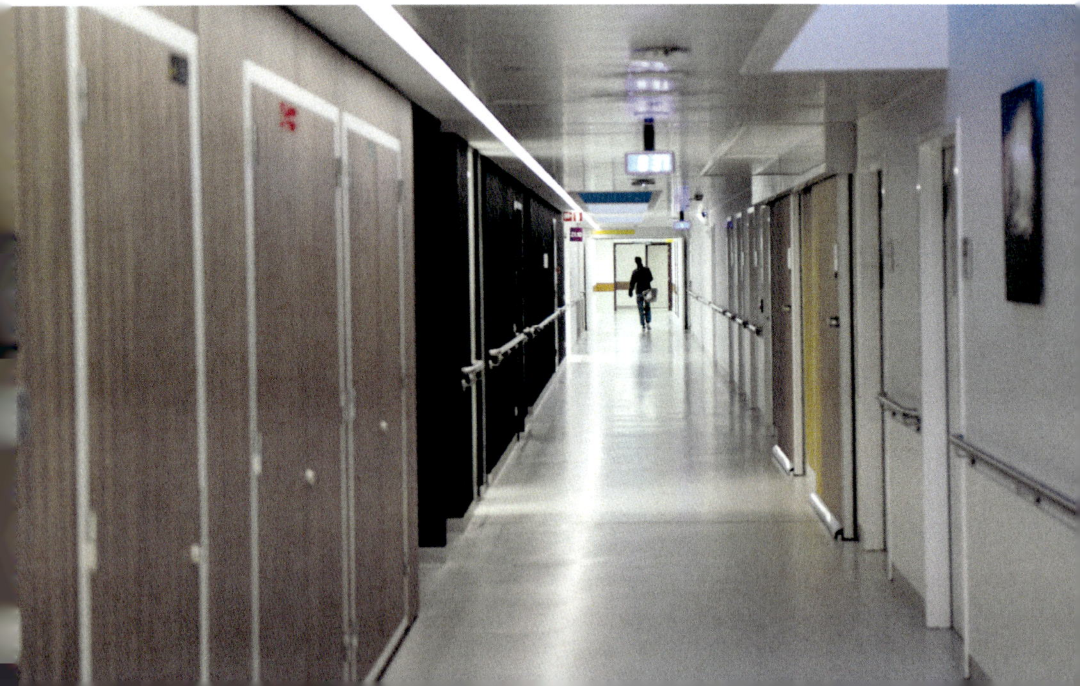

dealt with with every specific type of surgical intervention, compounded by patients own response to anesthetic medications.

Over time, this accumulates residue. The memory of near-misses. The weight of decisions made between imperfect options. The knowledge that a different choice, minutes earlier or later, could have altered the patient's outcome. These moments rarely make it into charts, but they settle quietly into the professional memory.

Burnout in anesthesiology feels like numbness. Going through motions without engagement. It looks like a narrowing of perspective, doing mechanically what is required, avoiding what once gave meaning. The specialty demands immense emotional regulation as a survival skill. You learn to contain fear, distraction, and personal concerns because the patient in front of you requires full presence. But containment is not elimination. What is set aside must eventually be addressed, or it leaks out elsewhere.

So how do anesthesiologists recover?

Some of us decompress physically, through sport, movement, exertion that restores a sense of control and embodiment. Others turn to music, art, writing, photography, hobbies-ways of processing without words what cannot easily be spoken. Some need silence. A time in the garden. Sharpness of mind is preserved by stepping away deliberately.

They cultivate interests that have nothing to do with medicine.

Teaching is a quiet form of renewal. Experience, when held alone, can feel heavy; its lessons learned

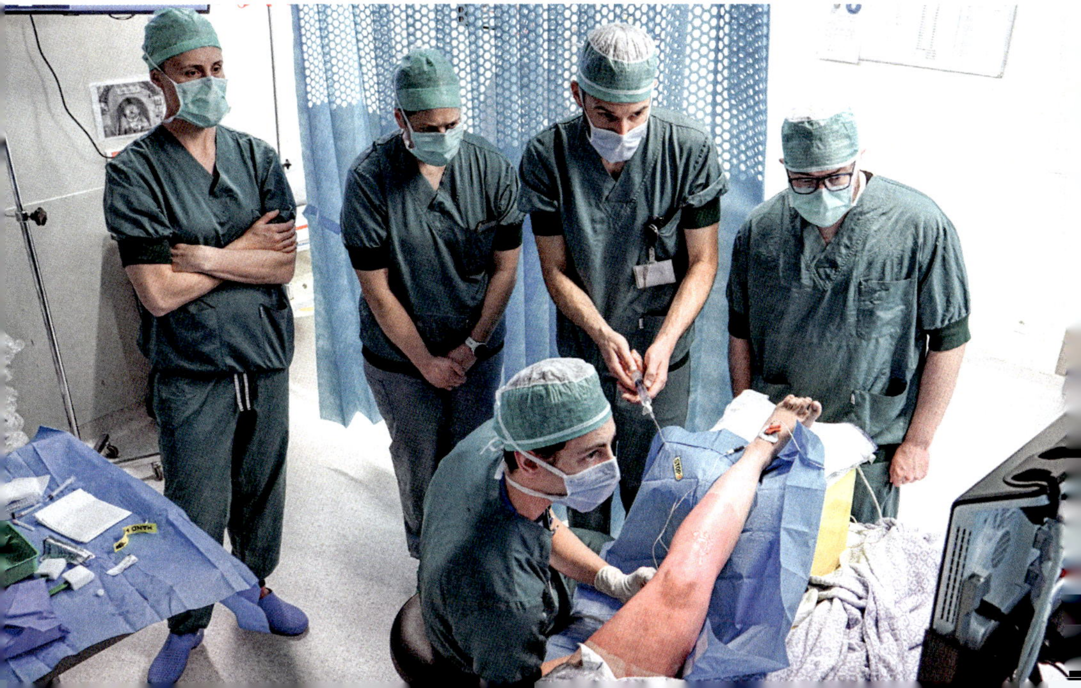

through strain, responsibility, and consequence. But when knowledge is passed forward, that weight begins to change. Moments once endured in isolation are given shape and purpose. Guiding others through paths you once walked alone transforms survival into continuity. What you carry is no longer just a burden of memory; it becomes something offered, something that outlives you, something that gives the work meaning again.

There is also honesty.

At some point, we all stop pretending that resilience means invulnerability. We more openly speak more openly about fatigue. About the need for boundaries. A culture that acknowledges limits is safer than one that denies them.

Anesthesiology asks a great deal. And that demand is amplified in moments of crisis: massive trauma cases, devastating accidents, pandemics like COVID. Those who endure are not the ones who ignore fatigue, but the ones who learn to hold the line between professional responsibility and a life beyond the hospital.

As one of my colleagues and lifelong inspirations, Dr. Jerry Vloka, once said, "If it were easy, everyone would do it." Anesthesiology is not for everyone, and those drawn to it must be certain they are prepared to carry responsibility when there is no margin for error.

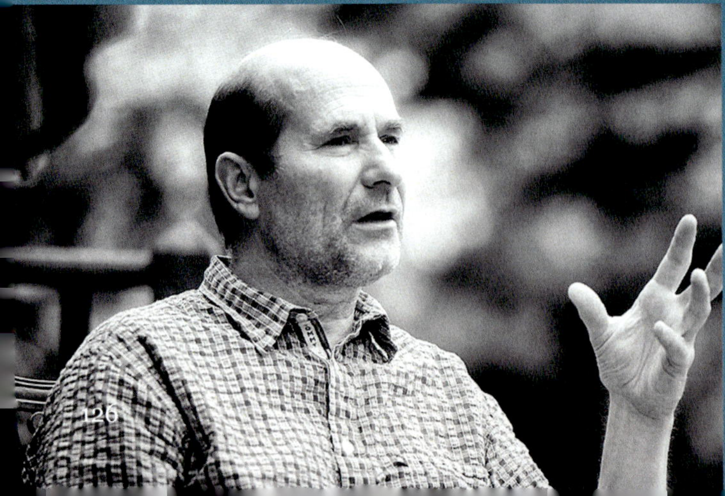

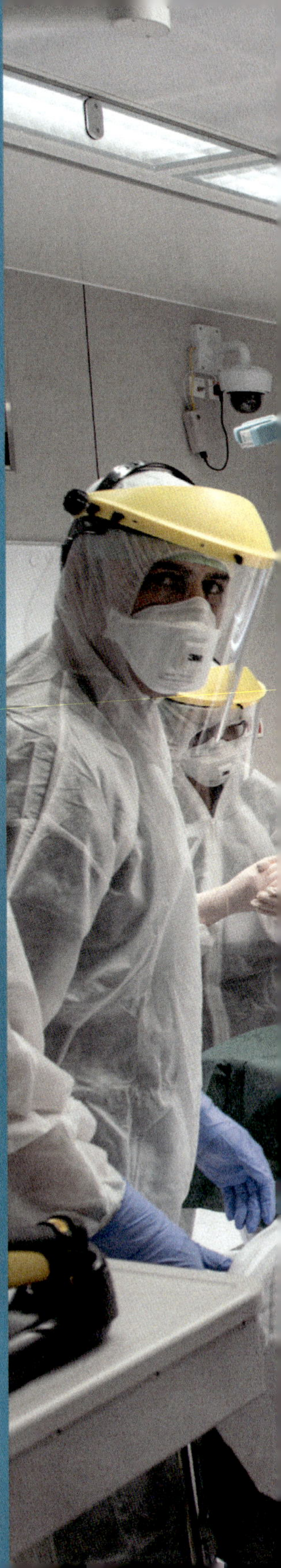

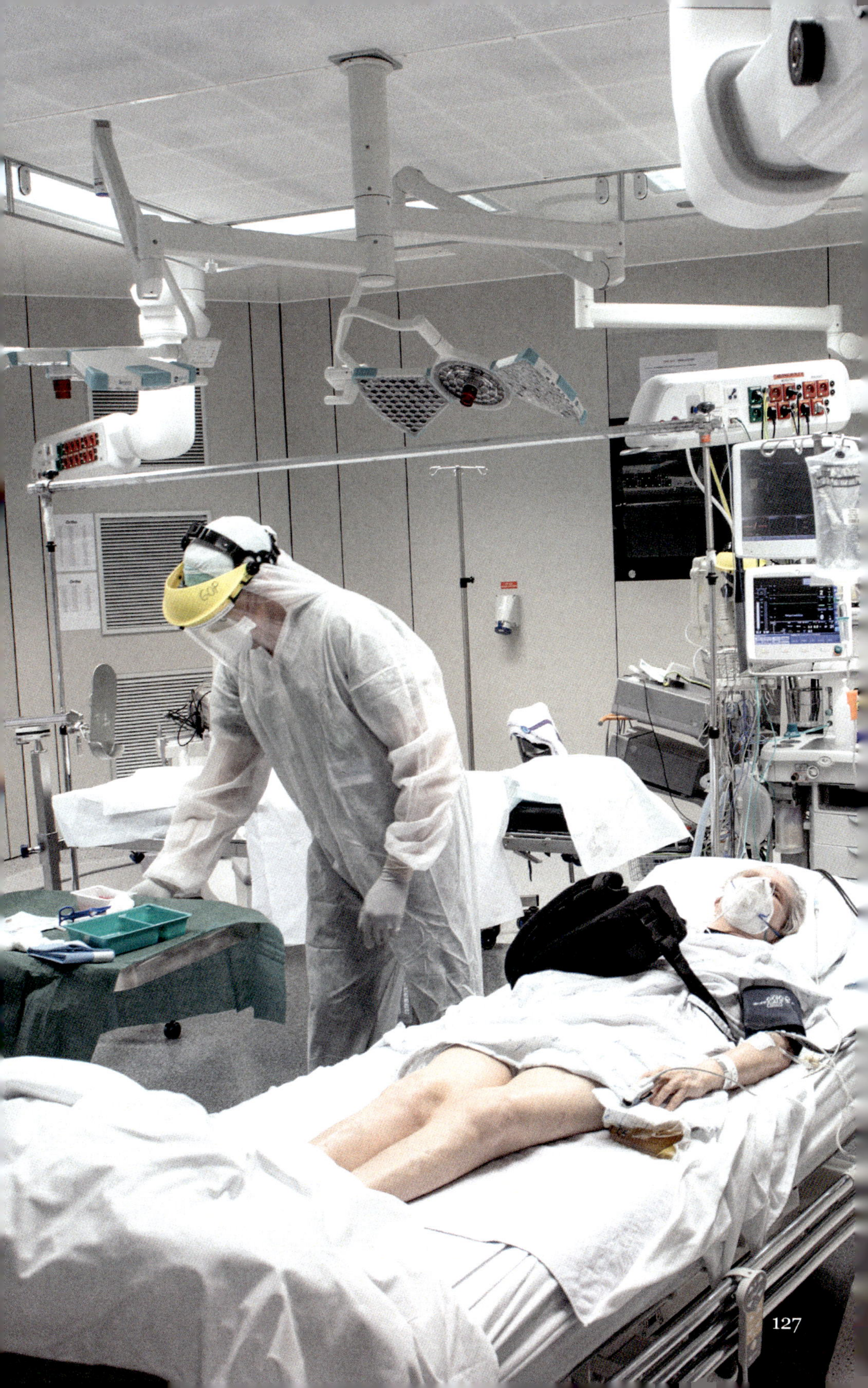

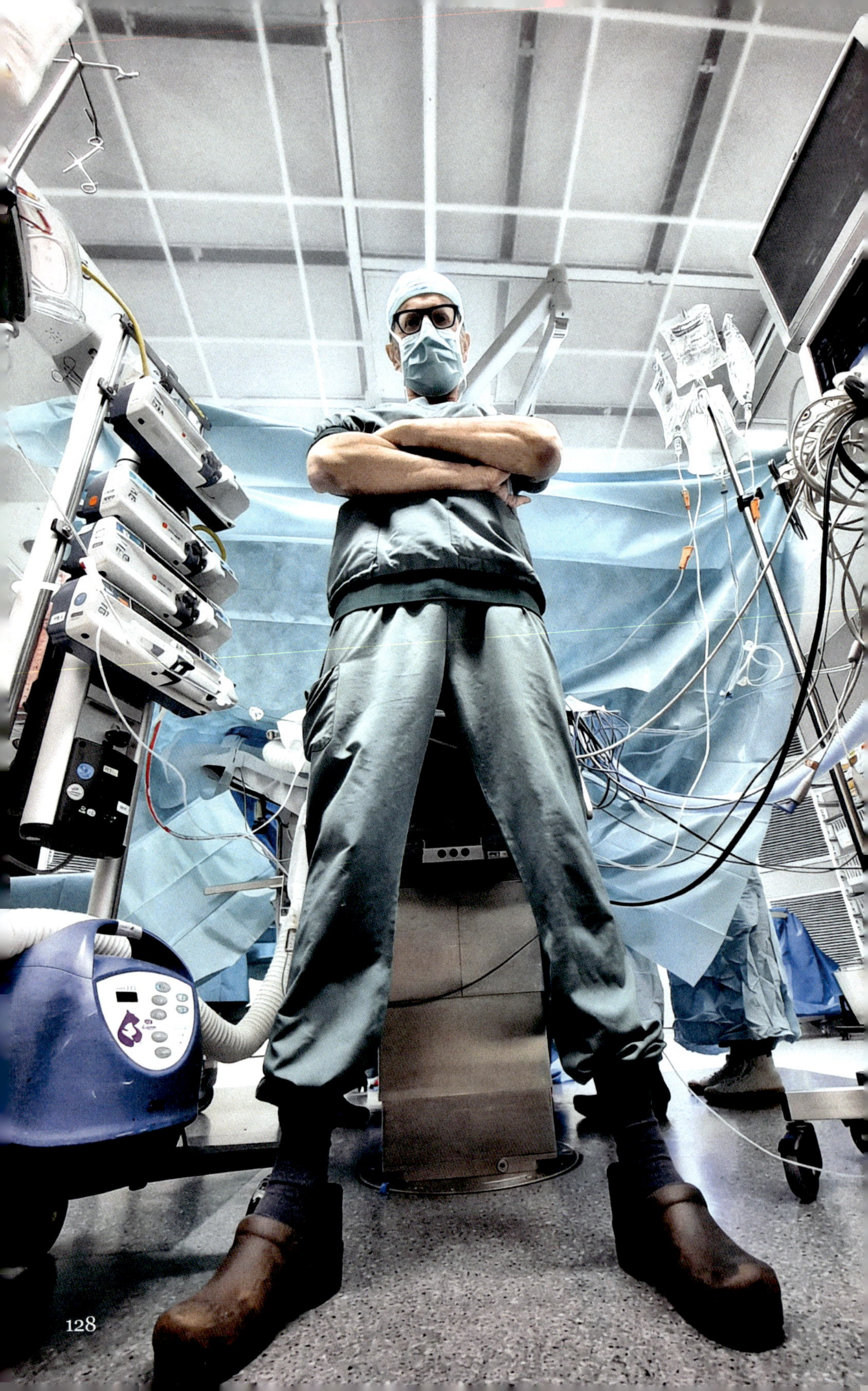

PART V

THE PROFESSION OVER TIME

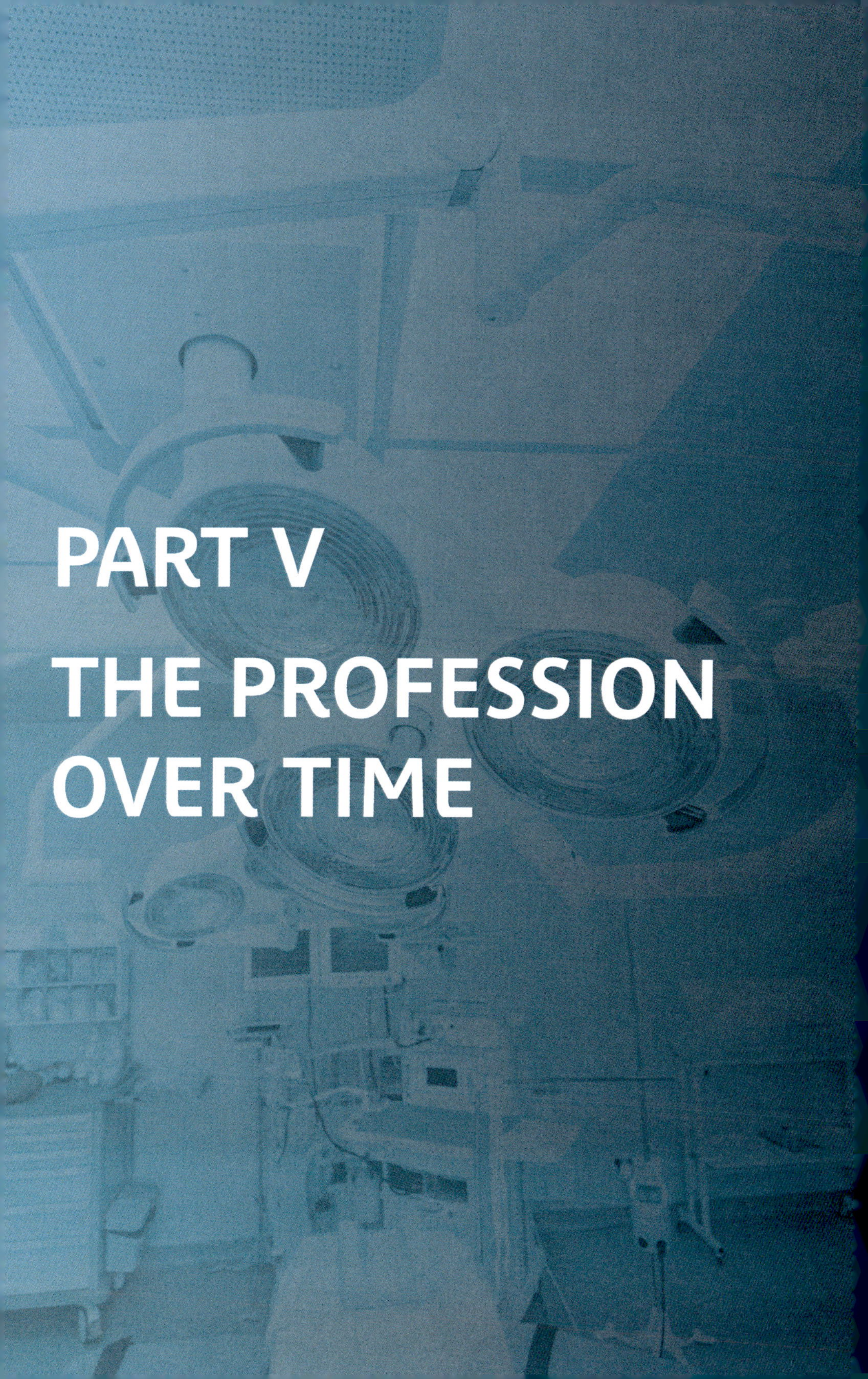

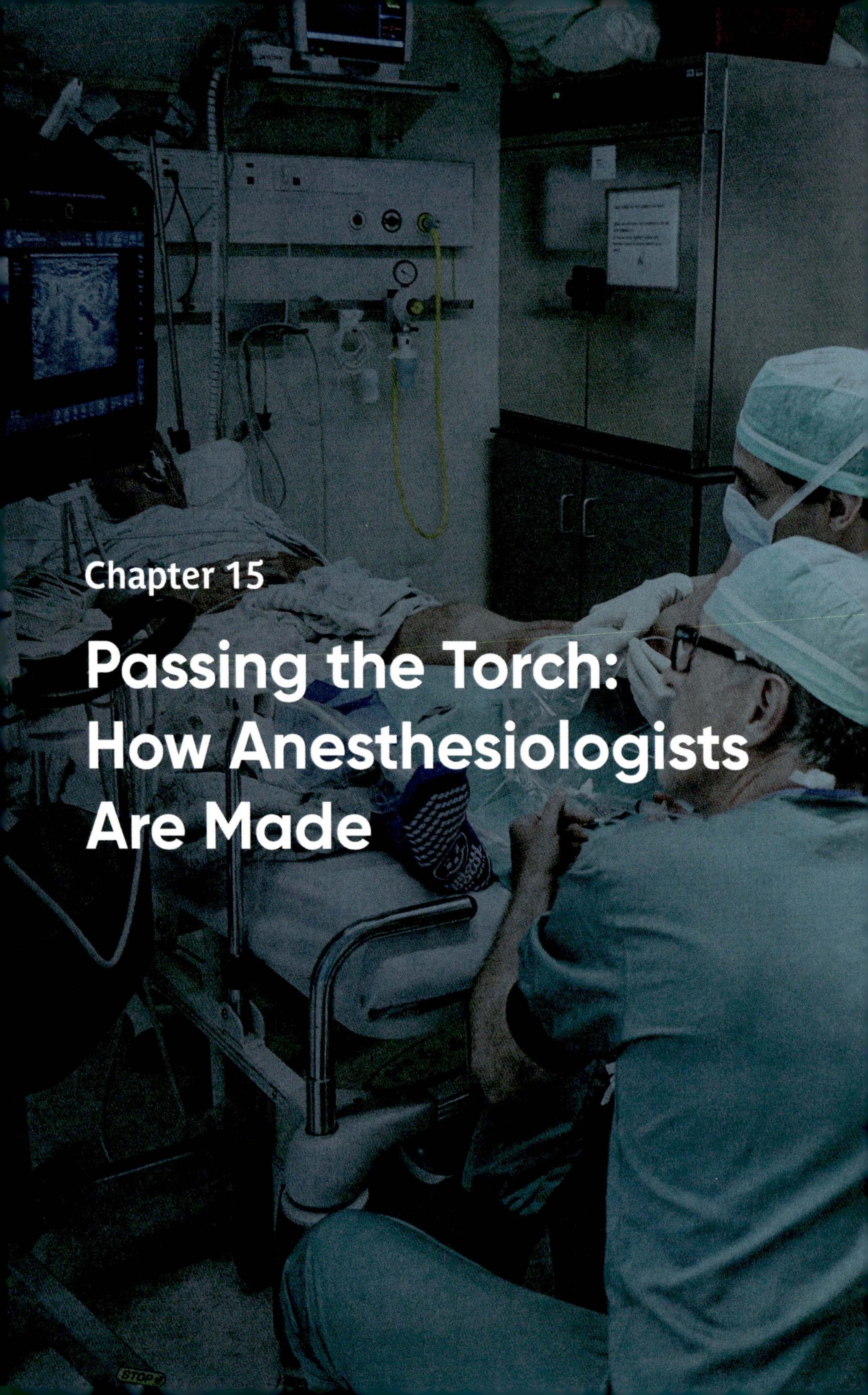

Chapter 15

Passing the Torch: How Anesthesiologists Are Made

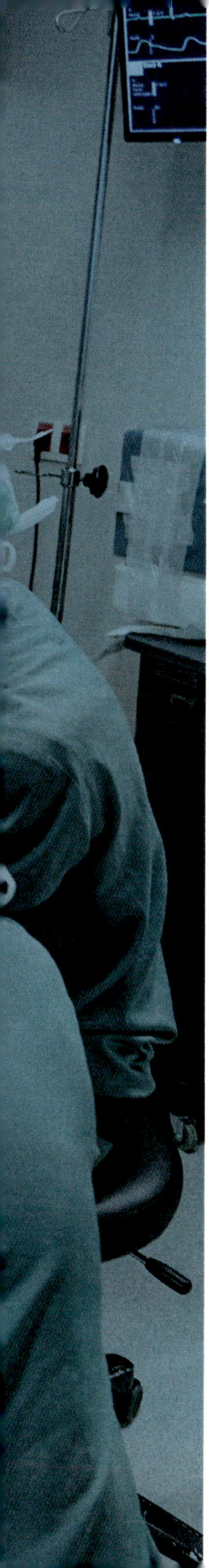

What matters most in the practice of anesthesiology can't be fully taught in classrooms or books. It's learned by watching and working along with experienced doctors at work. By seeing how they stay calm when things start to go wrong. How they prepare so well that problems are less likely to happen. How they notice danger before alarms start to beep.

This is how anesthesiologists are made. Not by lectures, but by example; one generation quietly teaching the next. Trainees who struggle, do so not because they lack intelligence, but because medicine often teaches complexity before clarity. We bury fundamentals under layers of information. We reward memorization instead of understanding. And then we wonder why young clinicians feel overwhelmed at the head of the bed. Anesthesiology does not forgive confusion; it rewards structure, repetition, and consistency.

The most effective teaching I have seen follows a simple arc: See-Do-Teach. It starts first by seeing excellence, then doing it under guidance, and then teaching it to someone else. That last step matters more than most realize. Teaching exposes gaps you didn't know you had. It humbles you. And it refines your craft in ways no theoretical course ever could.

I have seen the moment it clicks. A trainee stands at the head of the bed, and for the first time their eyes stop darting. Their hands slow down. Their voice steadies. They stop reacting to numbers and start understanding clinical trends. It's subtle, but to a teacher it is unmistakable: the real expertise has begun to form.

Clear visuals and standardized approaches are more reliable than improvisation. When techniques are structured, outcomes improve. When expectations are consistent, confidence follows.

Leading NYSORA has made this my responsibility: reducing complexity in education of anesthesiology, favoring structure, and teaching through visuals that endure. It is how knowledge survives, and how patients are protected.

The goal of education is not to create replicas of teachers. It is to create clinicians who can think independently within a reliable framework.

Perhaps the most rewarding moments of my career have not come from dramatic resuscitations or complex cases, but from quieter observations: a former trainee managing a difficult anesthetic case with calm precision. Or another teaching others with clarity; a young anesthesiologist recognizing danger early and preventing a crisis that never appears in a chart. In those moments, you know the torch has been passed.

Anesthesiology is a specialty built on continuity. Each generation inherits not only knowledge, but the responsibility to protect patients, respect physiology, and leave the discipline stronger than it was found.

And when you see your trainees take that responsibility, you know that the future of the specialty is in good hands, and the knowledge has been successfully passed onto the next generation of Life Savers.

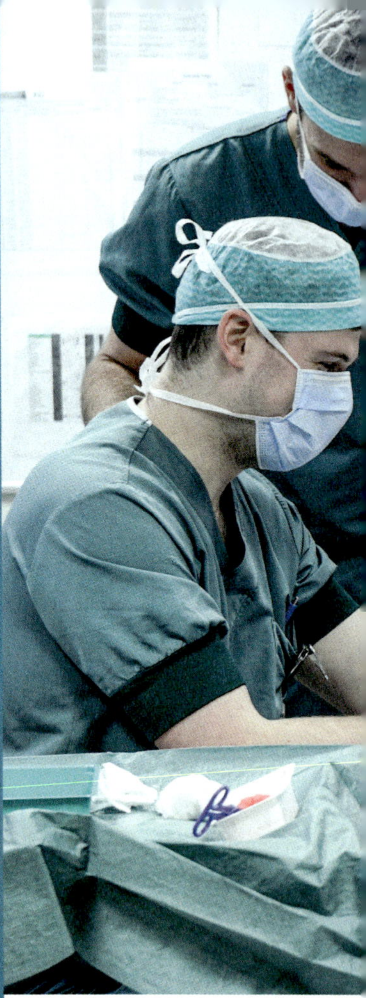

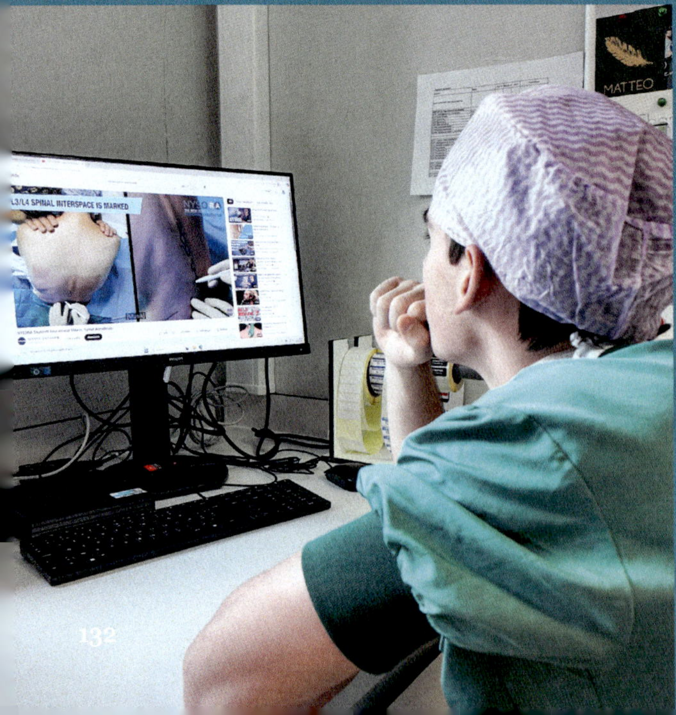

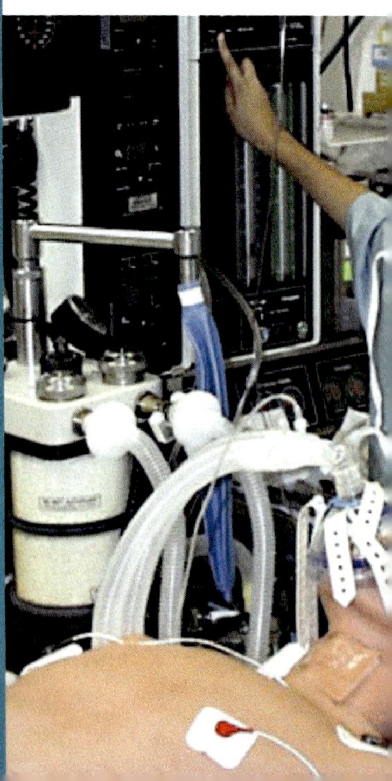

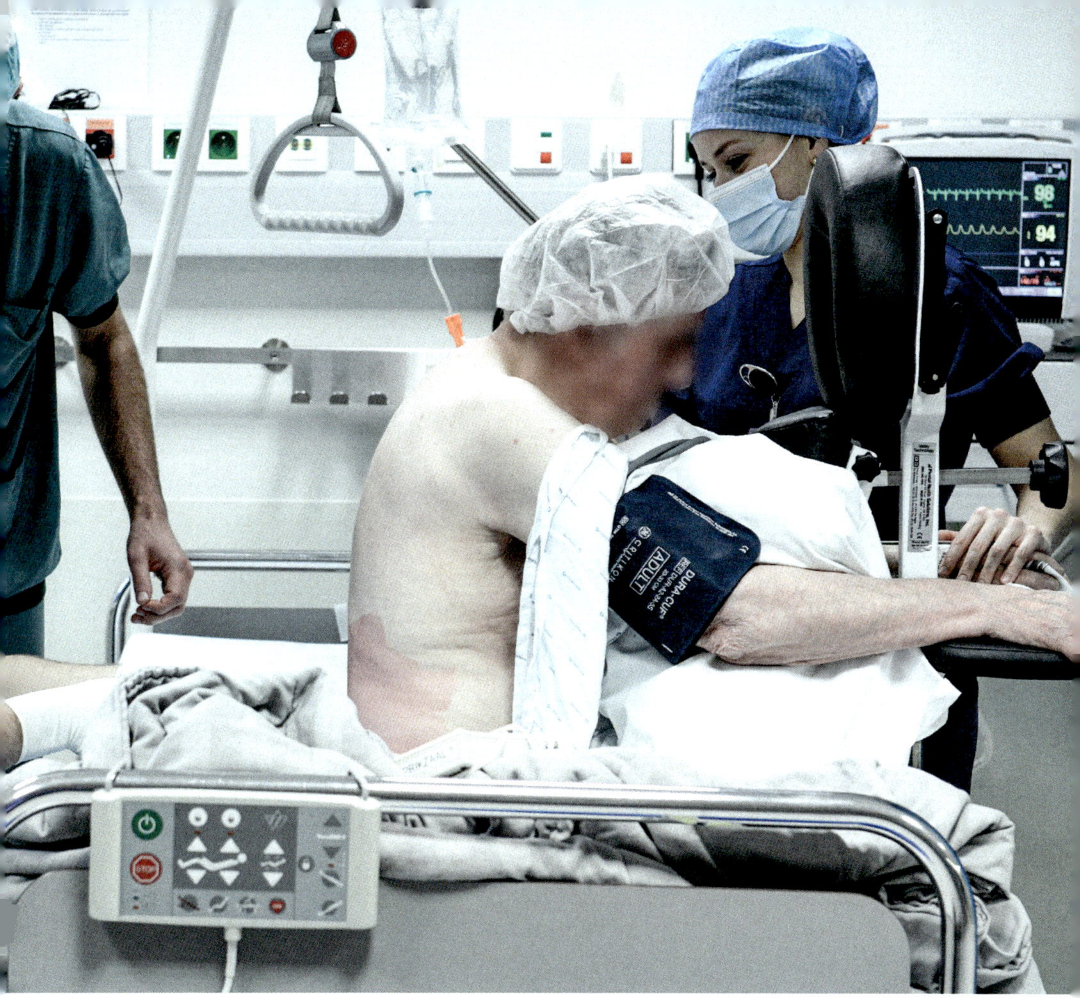
98
94
DURA-CUF
ADULT

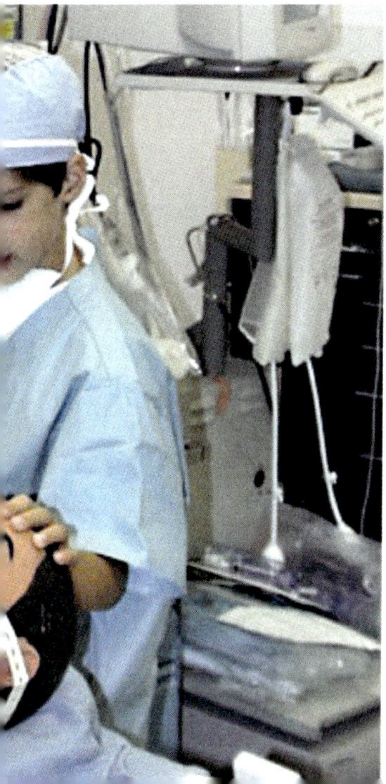

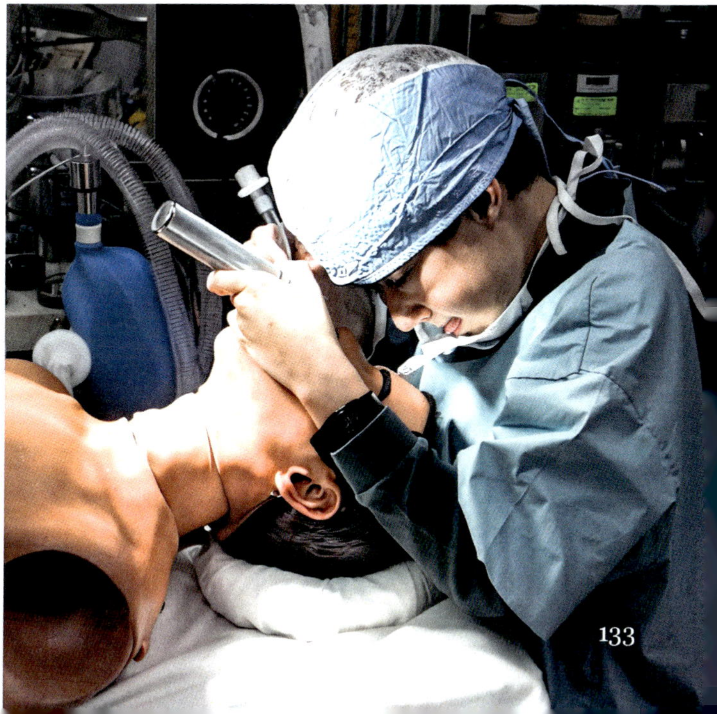

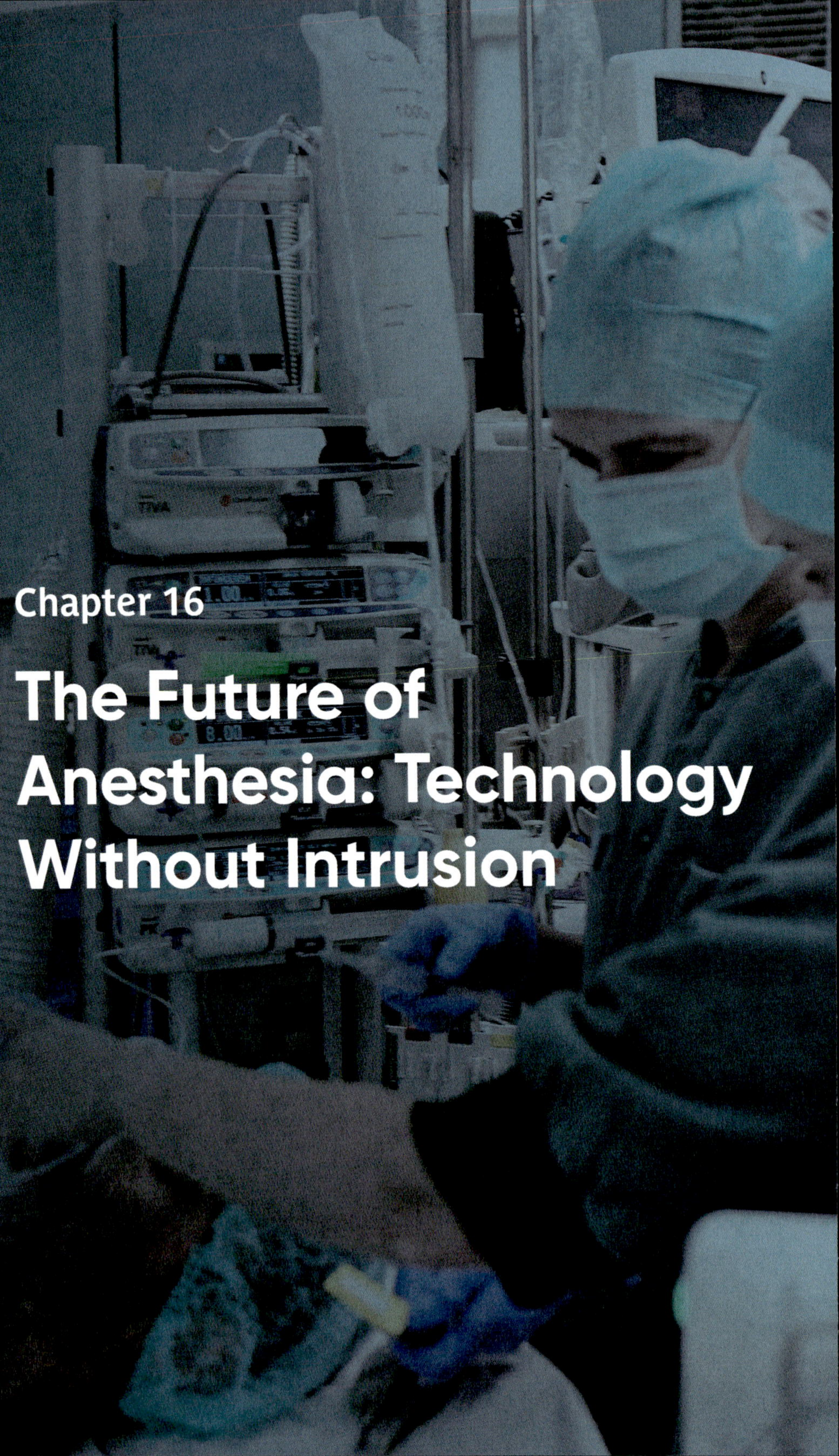

Chapter 16

The Future of Anesthesia: Technology Without Intrusion

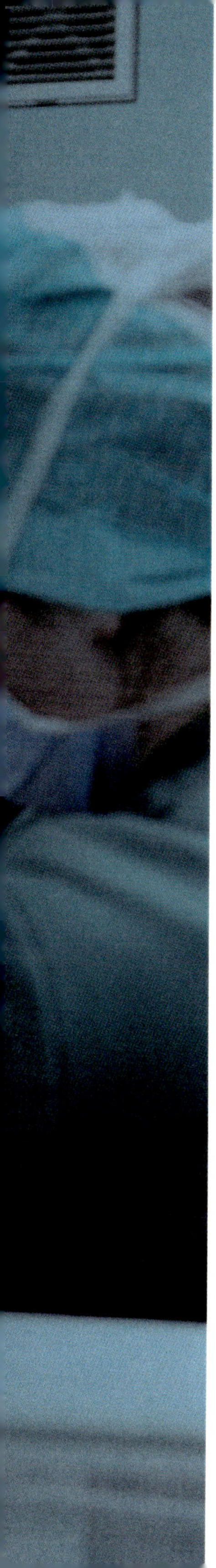

There is a quiet moment before every anesthetic. It comes after the equipment check and before anesthesia induction, after preparation, before action. The room is ready. The patient is awake. The team is aligned. Nothing dramatic is happening, yet everything that matters is about to.

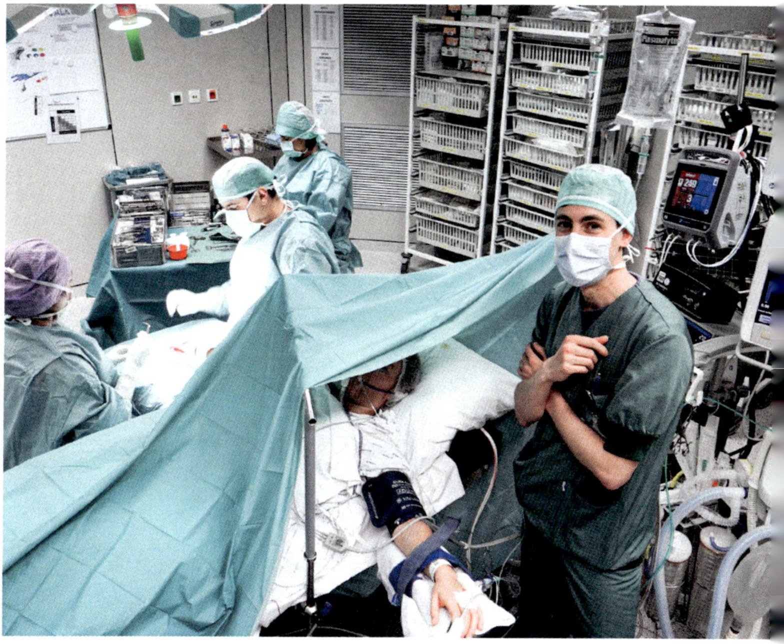

That moment has shaped how I think about technology in anesthesiology. Because anesthesia does not tolerate distraction; instead, it has always benefited from thoughtful innovation.

Few fields in medicine have been transformed as profoundly by technology as anesthesiology. Monitoring, imaging, pharmacology, airway devices, portable ultrasound systems, and safety systems have made our work measurably safer, more predictable, and more humane. Mortality has fallen. Complications are anticipated earlier. Margins of safety that once depended entirely on experience are now supported by data.

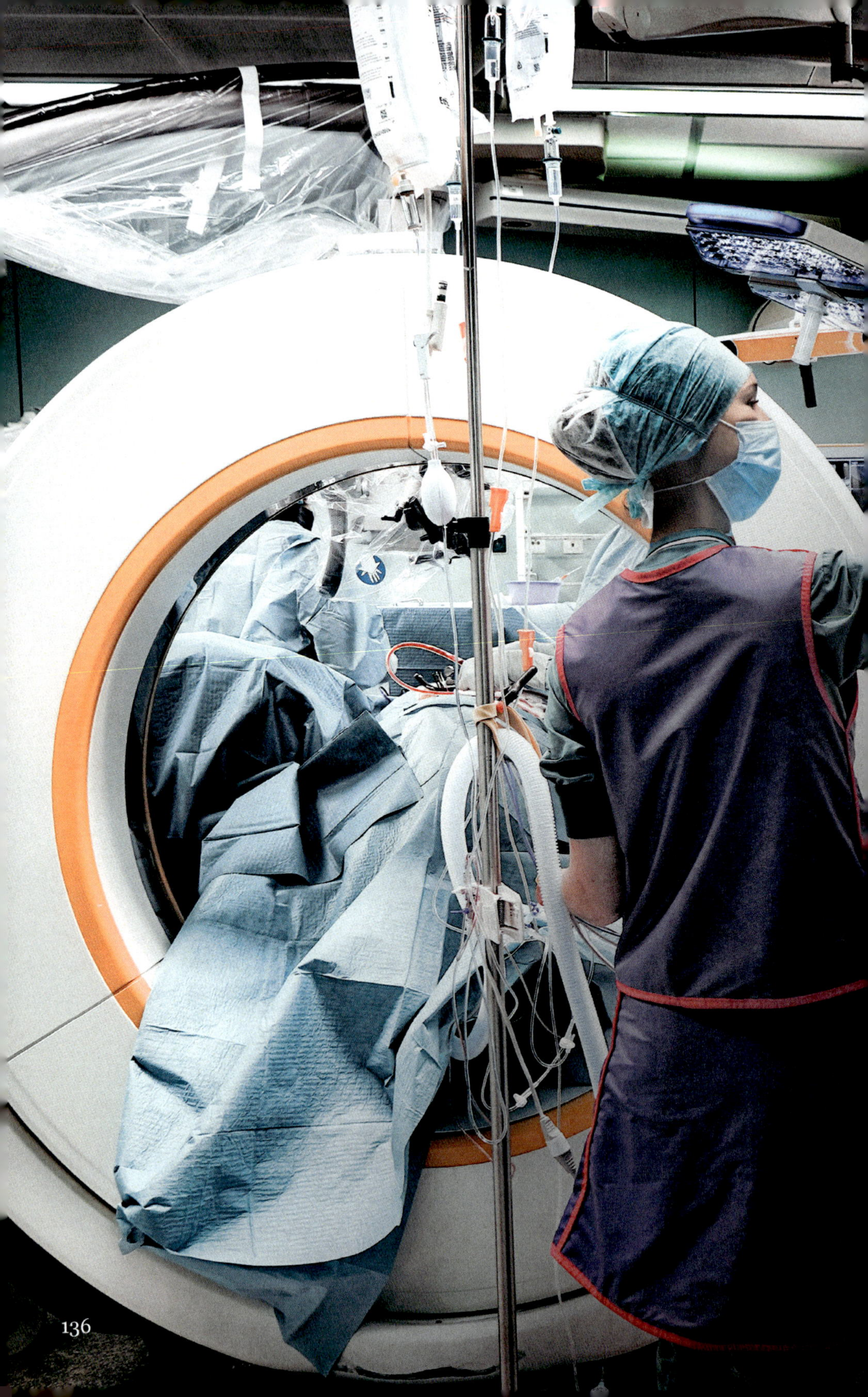

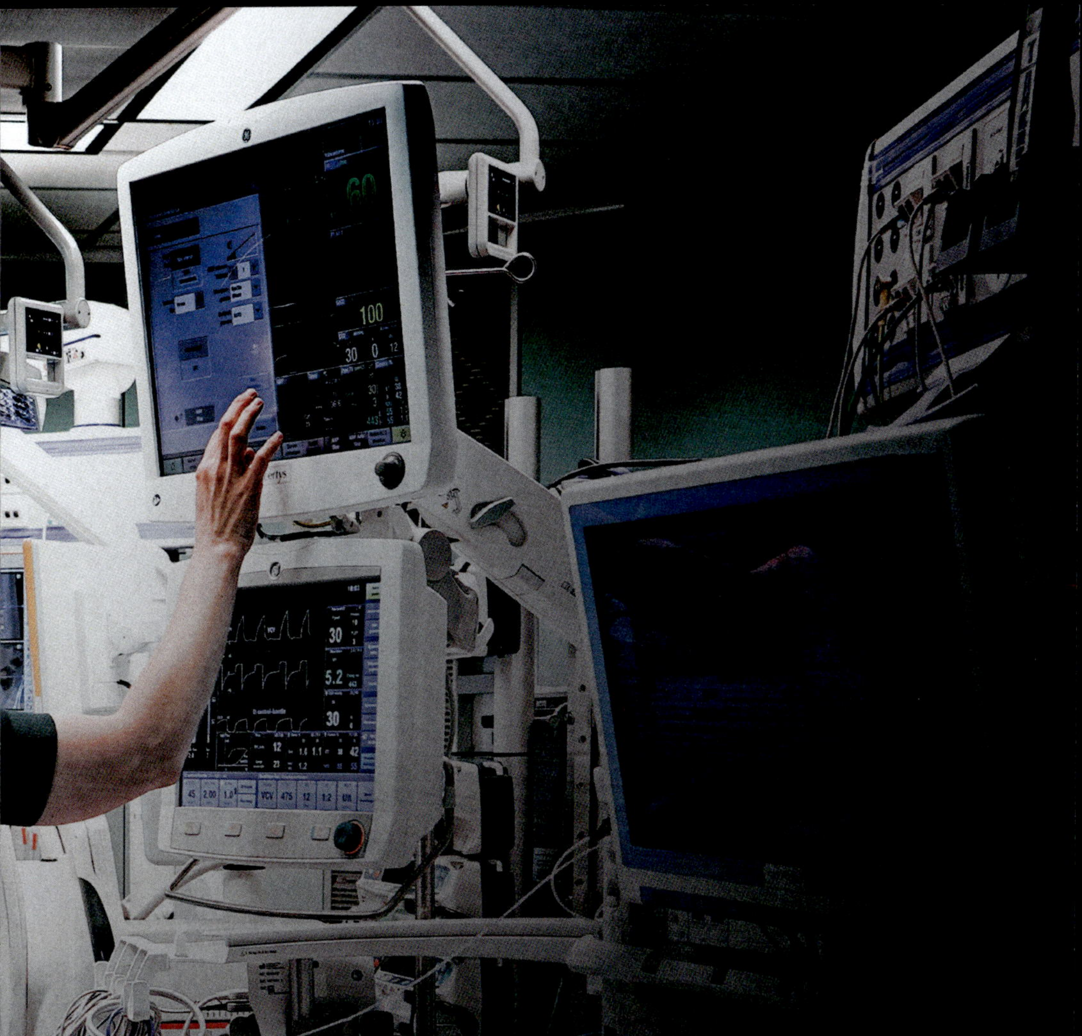

Technology has earned its place at the head of the bed. But how it integrates in our work flow matters.

Anything that competes for attention at that critical instant, anything that demands unnecessary clicks, confirmations, or interruptions, must be carefully reconsidered. Anesthesiology is not short on information. It is short on margin. And the difference between help and harm often lies in whether a tool supports judgment or distracts from it.

I remember standing at the head of the bed during a routine case when a new automated monitoring system we just installed in the hospital chimed insistently, alerting me to something I already knew and had already addressed. The patient was stable. The alert demanded acknowledgment, as if attention itself were a checkbox.

I silenced it. Not because technology was wrong, but because in that moment, it was poorly timed. Anesthesiologists have never been anti-technology. But we have always been critical and selective.

We have lived through waves of innovation: advanced monitors, sophisticated airway tools, smarter alarms, electronic records. All intended to streamline care. Many of these advances have positively contributed to safety of anesthesia. Others have added friction without benefit, such as cacophony of endless alarms that require constant reset, recalibration and may be more distractive than helpful in the clinical practice. What ultimately endures are tools that respect workflow, context, and clinical judgment that do their work without demanding to be noticed.

Anesthesiology does not need technology to lead. It needs technology to support the clinicians. The future of our specialty will not be defined by machines or AI replacing clinicians, but by systems that facilitate routine decision-making so that human judgment is preserved for moments that truly require it. The best technology in anesthesia reduces cognitive load rather than adds to it. It standardizes what should be standard, so that attention is freed for what cannot be standardized.

This distinction matters especially as

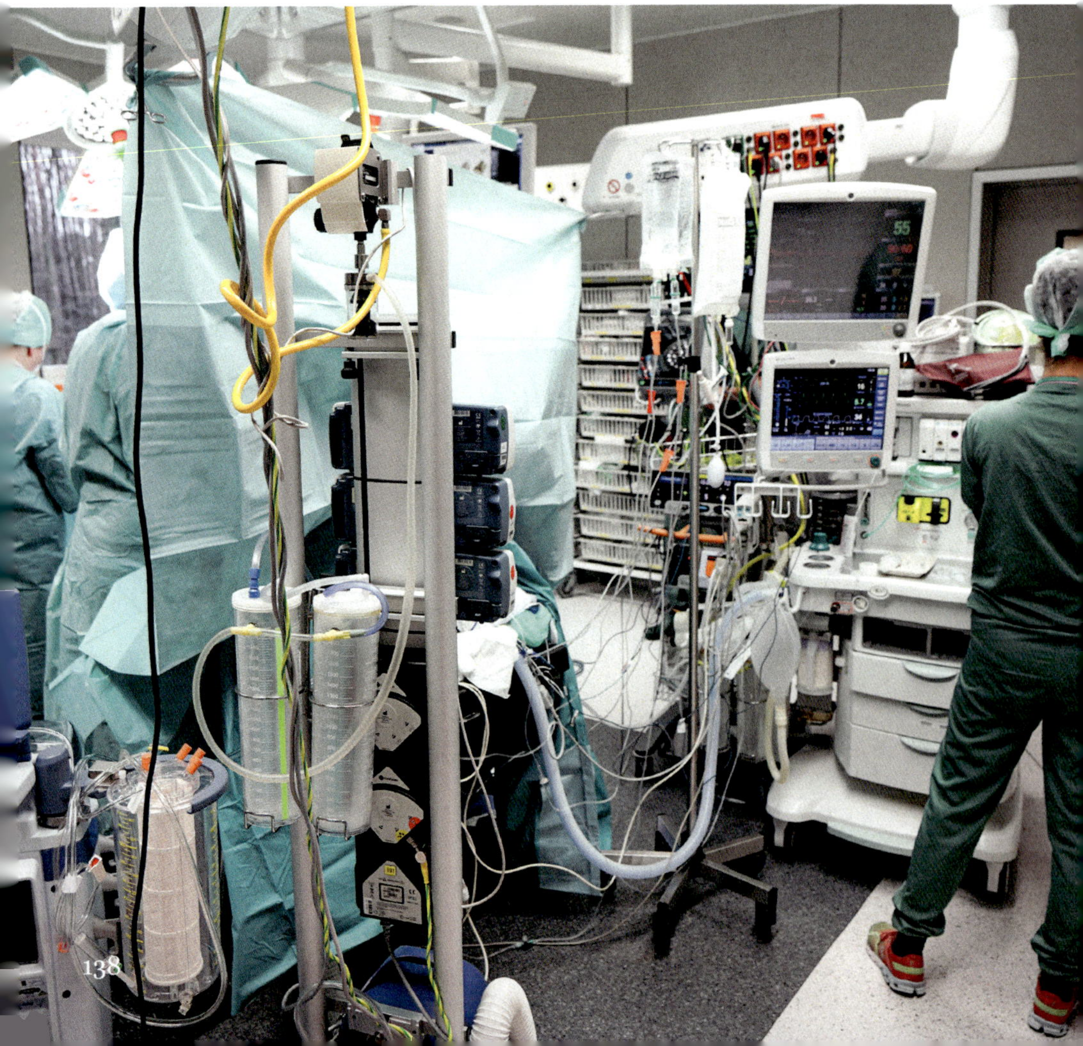

artificial intelligence enters the clinical space. AI is no longer theoretical. It is here, and it is advancing rapidly. However, used carelessly, it risks becoming another source of noise. Used well, it holds a real promise particularly in education, and structured clinical thinking.

AI tools such as NYSORA's Anesthesia Assistant App, point toward this future supported by AI that leans on peer-reviewed information. Not as a replacement for clinical presence, but as a platform for case discussions, simulations, and time-efficient patient management review. This is where AI fits naturally: helping clinicians think better, prepare better, and reflect more deeply without competing for attention when seconds matter. In anesthesia, the best tools feel almost invisible. They do not announce themselves. They do not interrupt the quiet moment before induction. They wait. They support.

At the head of the bed, there will still be a human being, carrying the responsibility that no algorithm can assume.

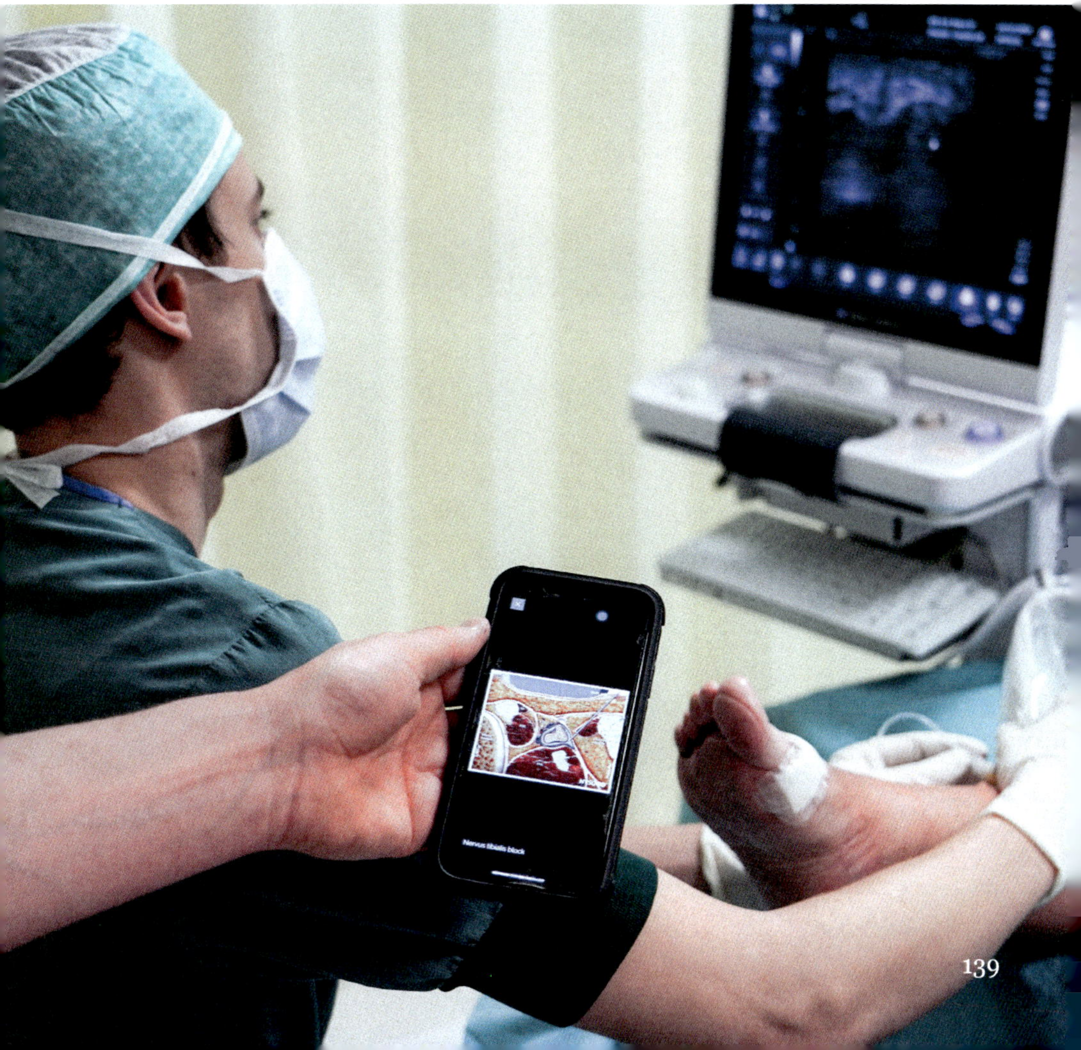

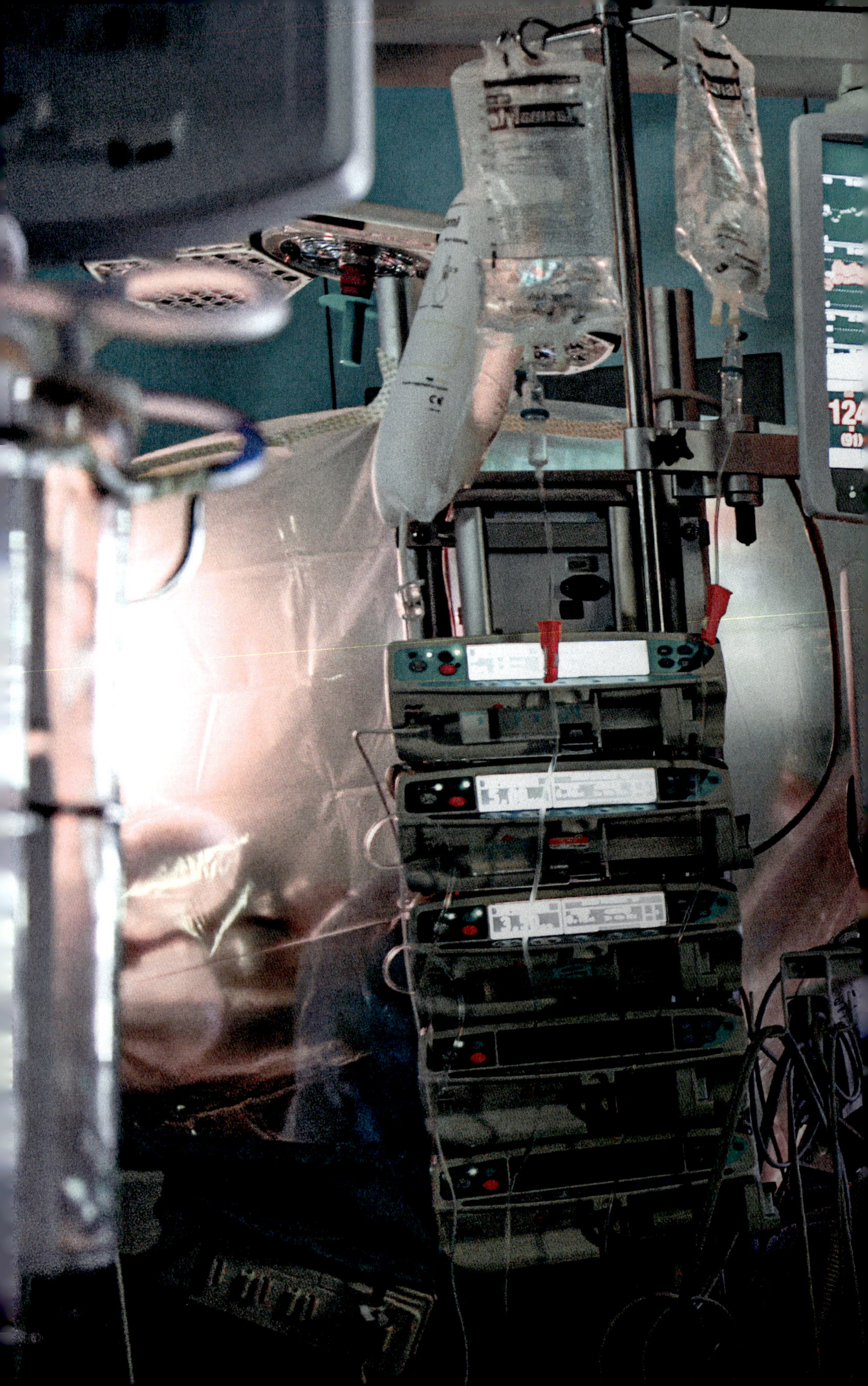
124
(91)

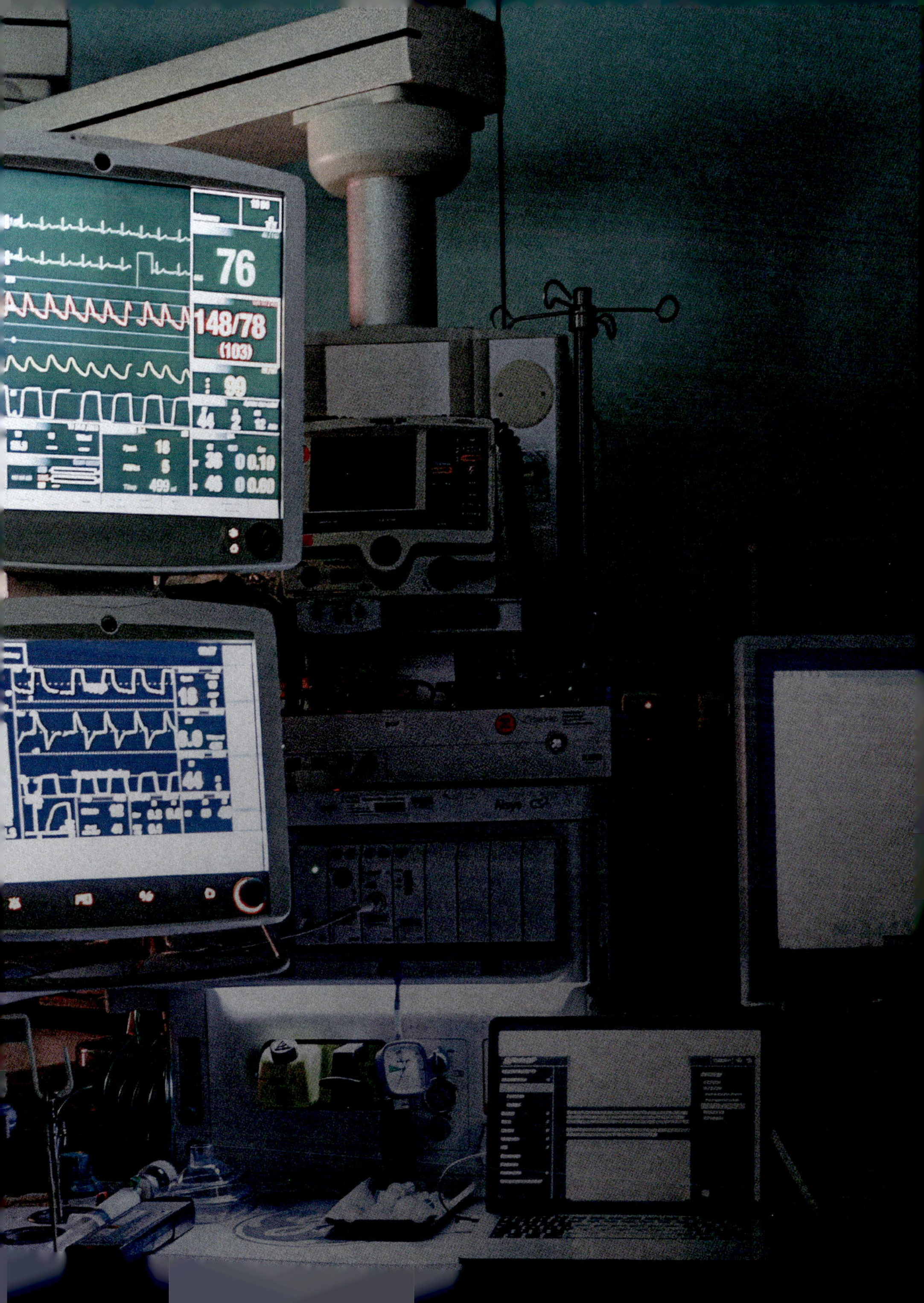
76
148/78
(103)

Chapter 17

Should You Become an Anesthesiologist?

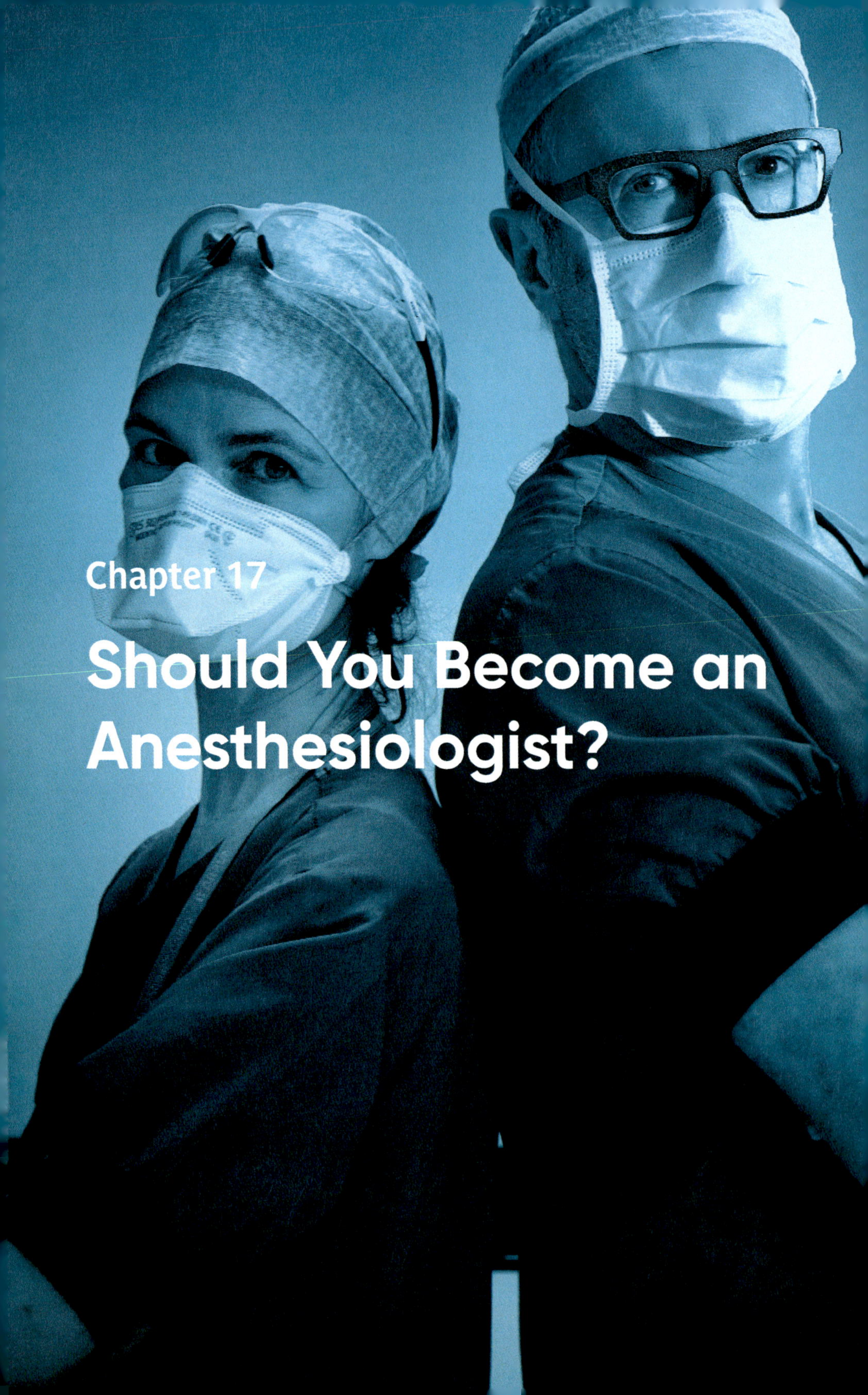

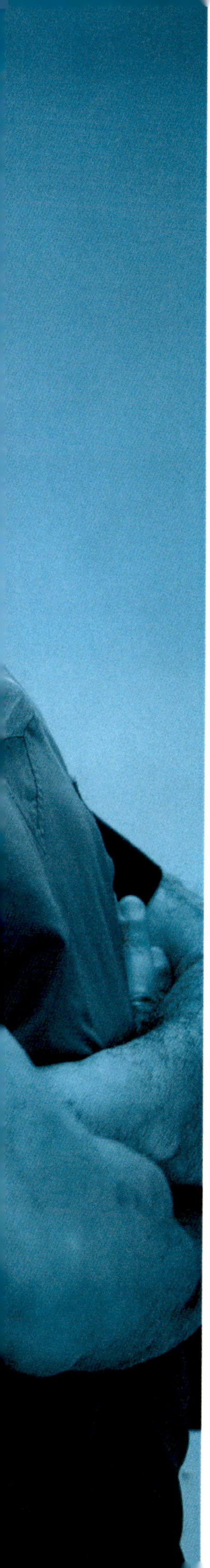

The Five Cs That Decide Everything

When students ask me whether they should become anesthesiologists, my answer often surprises them. I tell them the truth. It depends on two things: manual dexterity and the ability to remain calm and focused under constant multitasking stress. Everything else, including theoretical knowledge, can be learned more easily. In the OR, you have to be able to swim, or you sink.

The operating room is a place most people never truly see. Because of that, anesthesiology is often misunderstood. It is best understood by observing how anesthesiologists work, how they think, anticipate, and make decisions in real time. This book is meant to show that work as it actually happens. I choose anesthesiology as a profession after witnessing the work, the responsibility, and the moments when everything depends on one person staying calm and making the right decision. One night in particular, I described at the beginning of this book in “The Night That Changed Everything”- set that path in motion.

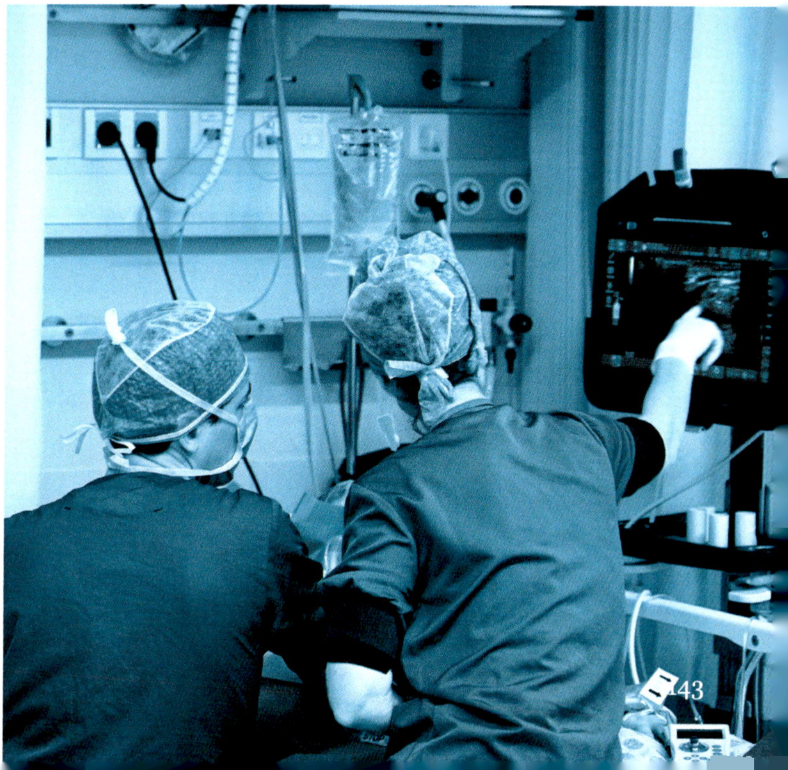

Skill in anesthesiology is never something you "finish" learning, and without manual confidence, no amount of theoretical knowledge can make the next unpredictable case feel manageable.

I remember a Columbia University student sitting across from me at St. Luke 's - Roosevelt Hospital in NYC, after a long, but uneventful day in the operating room. Smart. Motivated. Clearly capable. He had watched several easy, elective cases, asked good questions, and finally said, "I think I'd like anesthesia, it looks calm". He couldn't have been more mistaken. What he had seen was not the work, it was the silence between storms.

Over the years, I have come to believe that a great anesthesiologist must possess five essential character traits. Not four. Not three. All five.

If even one is missing, anesthesiology as a profession will be a lifelong struggle.

I call them the **Five Cs**.

1. COMMITMENT

Commitment is not the same as motivation.
Motivation depends on external rewards, recognition, praise, prestige. If that is what you are looking for, anesthesiology will disappoint you. The surgeon is the visible face of the operation, and rightly so; that is the role the patient recognizes.Commitment comes from within.
Commitment means showing up when no one is watching. It means preparing for cases that may never challenge you and being ready when one suddenly does. In anesthesiology, patients' lives depend on your mastery of the craft, not on how inspired you feel that morning.

2. COURAGE

From the moment you administer anesthesia, the patient's life is quite literally in your hands. Within minutes, a walking, talking human being becomes immobile, silent, and completely vulnerable, dependent on you to breathe, circulate blood, and survive.
That responsibility is immense. But it cannot paralyze you.
Fear may push others into panic. An anesthesiologist must remain calm, focused, and decisive. You must assess, anticipate, and act often under pressure, often without backup, and often without time to reflect.

There is no pause button.

There is no committee meeting.

There is no second opinion in real time.

3. CONFIDENCE

Confidence is not arrogance.
It is quiet preparedness.
Anesthesiology demands instant decision-making. If you prefer long deliberation, extended reflection, or consensus, building over hours

or days, this field will exhaust you. Here, decisions are made in seconds.

To function at that level without constant anxiety, your skills must be deeply etched, so familiar that they can be summoned without hesitation. Confidence comes from mastery, and mastery comes from repetition, reflection, and continuous learning.The moment you stop learning, confidence fades.

4. CONSISTENCY

Knowledge alone is not enough.

Anesthesiology is a hands-on craft. Manual dexterity matters. Hand-eye coordination matters. A steady hand matters.

This is not a specialty that tolerates improvisation disguised as skill. Like musicians practicing scales or athletes training fundamentals, anesthesiologists must practice continuously. Performance must be accurate, repeatable, and reliable, especially under pressure.

5. CHARISMA

This one surprises people.

An anesthesiologist must lead. And leadership requires charisma.

Charisma is not charm or theatrics. It is self-trust. When you trust yourself, others trust you. In the operating room, that trust aligns teams, sharpens communication, and creates calm when chaos threatens.

Charisma allows instructions to be followed instantly, without explanation, without hesitation.The Question Revisited

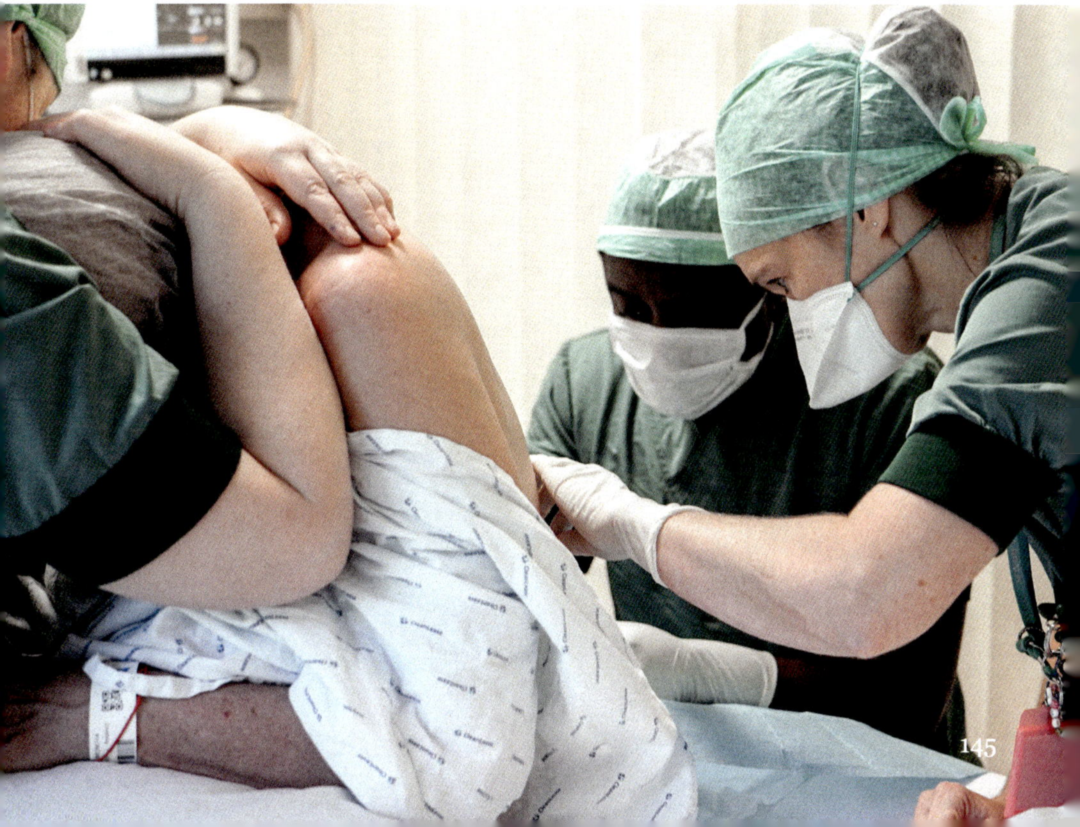

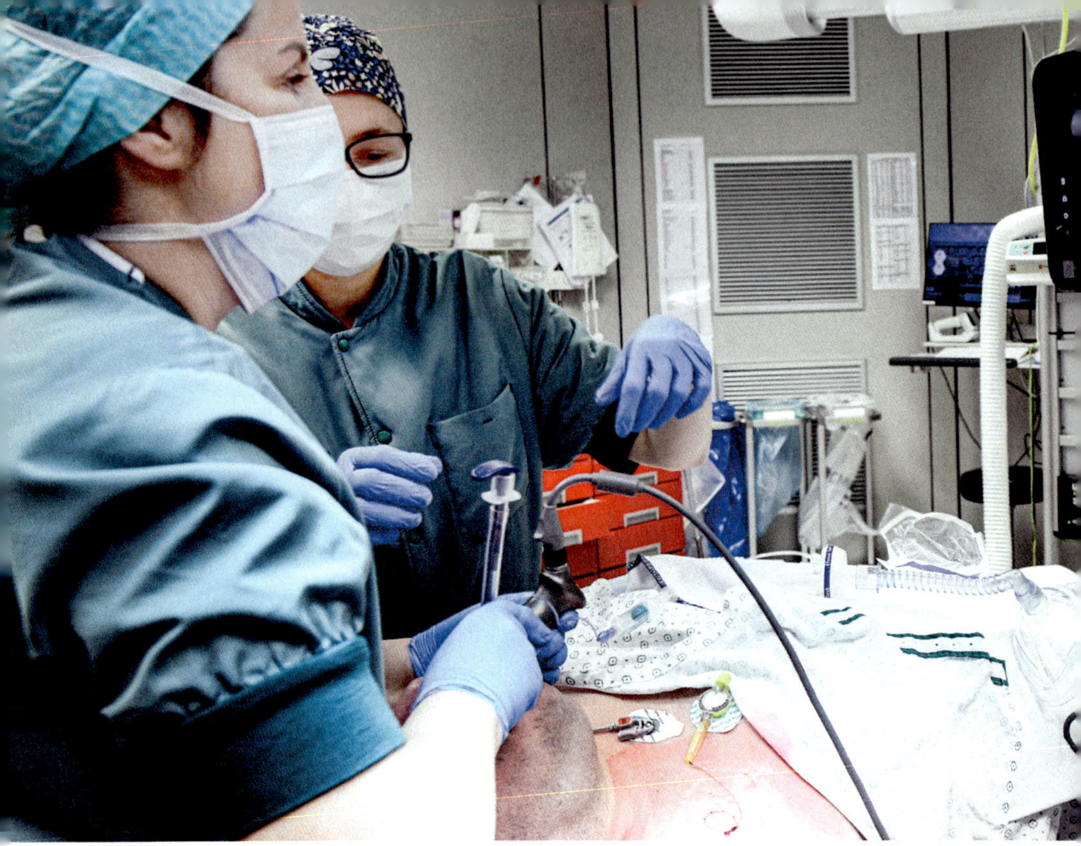

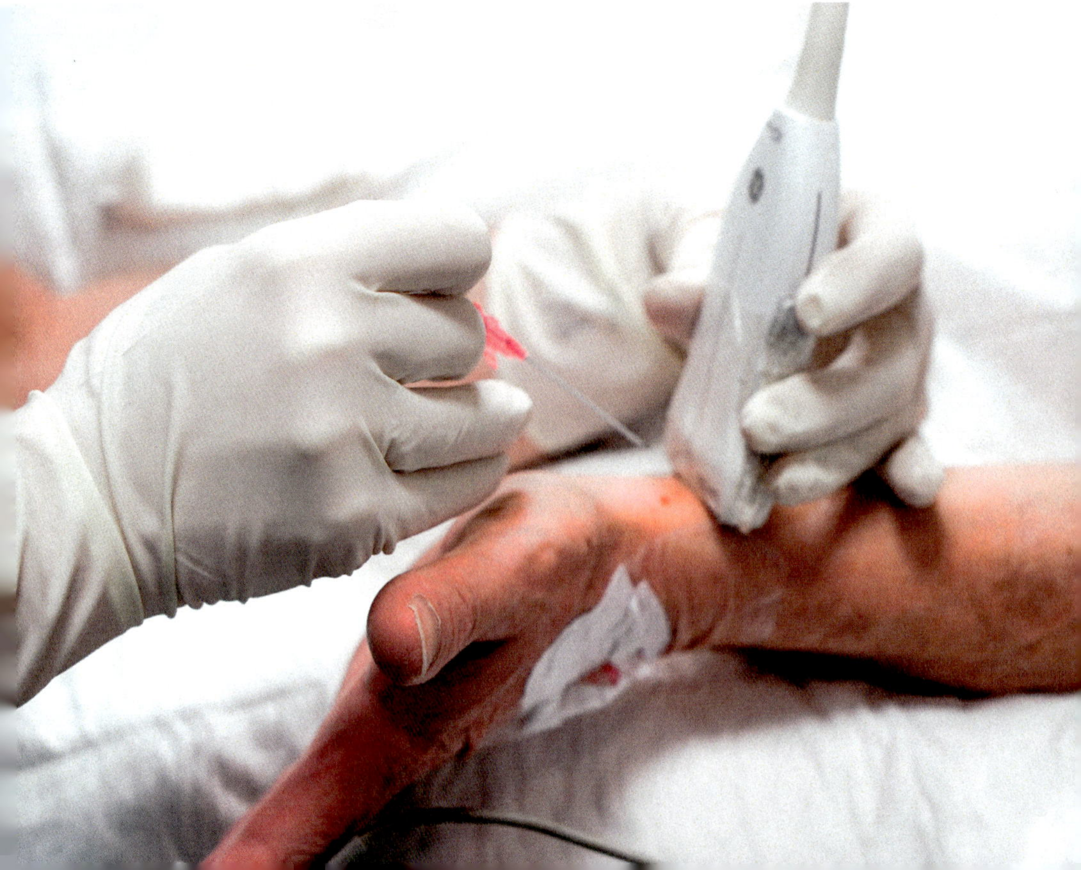

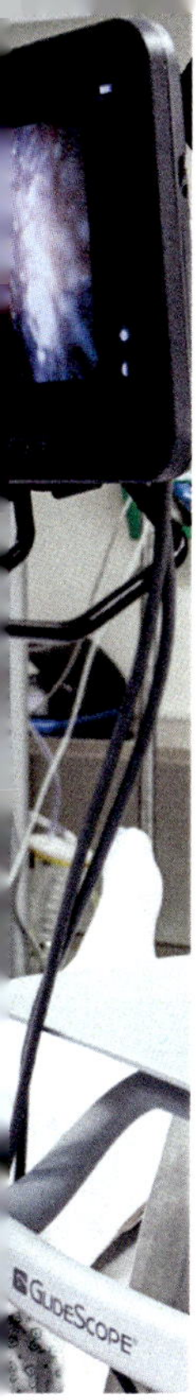
GlideScope
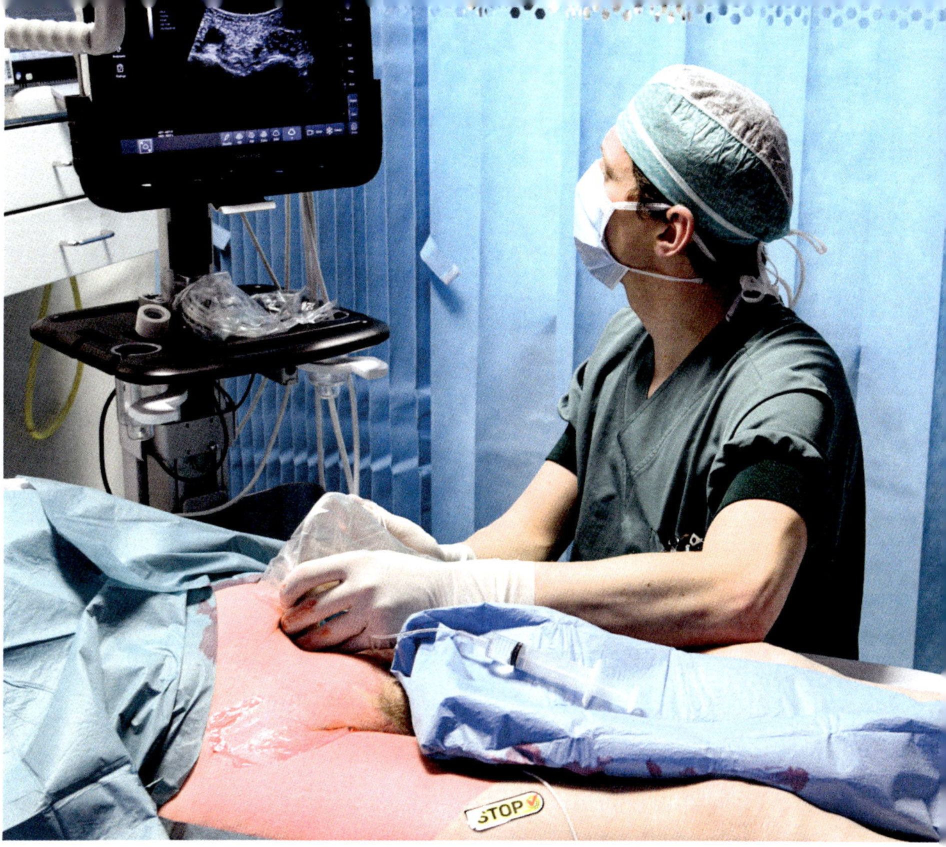
STOP

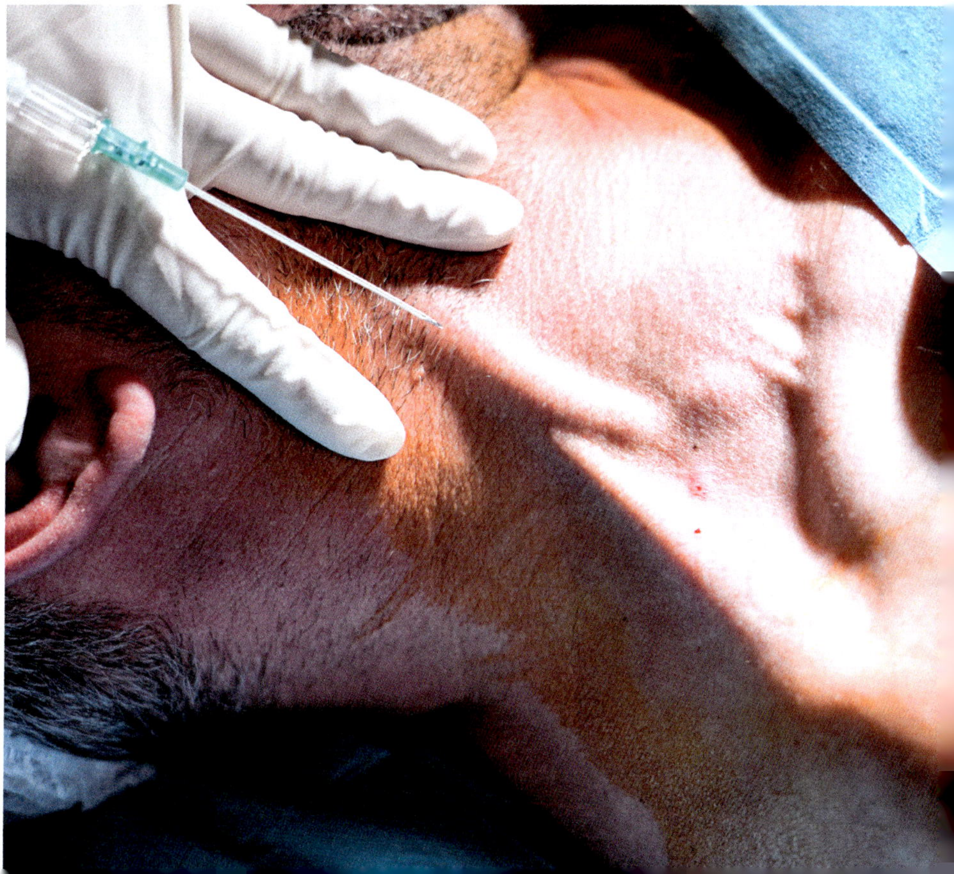

The Question Revisited

So, should you become an anesthesiologist?

Only if you have **commitment**, **courage**, **confidence**, **consistency**, and **charisma**.

Not some of them.

Not most of them.

All five.

If you are considering becoming an anesthesiologist, you should understand one thing early: you will rarely be in the spotlight. Surgeons receive most of the credit and rightly so, because patients come to the hospital for the operation itself, not for anesthesia. Anesthesiology happens in the background, and you must be comfortable working there in the rhythm section, without recognition or applause.

The role is much like the story told in the American documentary " Standing in the Shadows of Motown". The film reveals the Funk Brothers, the uncredited, extraordinarily skilled studio musicians behind the Motown sound, in Detroit, Michigan. Without them, the iconic music of artists like Michael Jackson, Stevie Wonder, Marvin Gaye, Smokey Robinson, and Diana Ross would not exist. Yet they remained largely unseen.

Anesthesiologists are that rhythm section. Leadership without spotlight. Precision without praise. The steady, positive energy that allows the headline act to succeed. Anesthesiology is not about glory. It is about responsibility.

When that student asked me if anesthesia was "calm," I told him the truth: it looks calm only when someone competent is working very hard to make it that way.

If that responsibility excites you rather than frightens you, then anesthesiology may not just be a career.

It may be your calling.

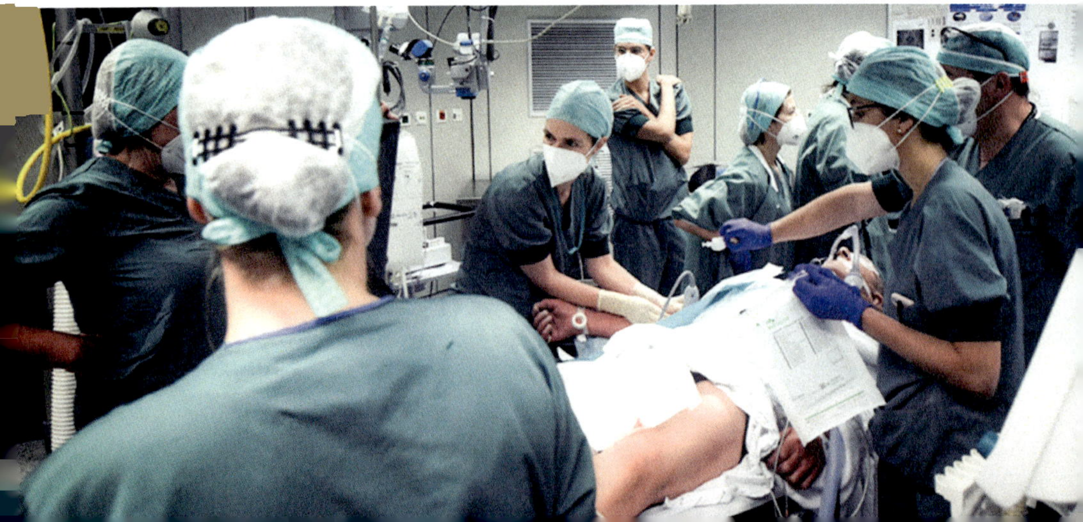

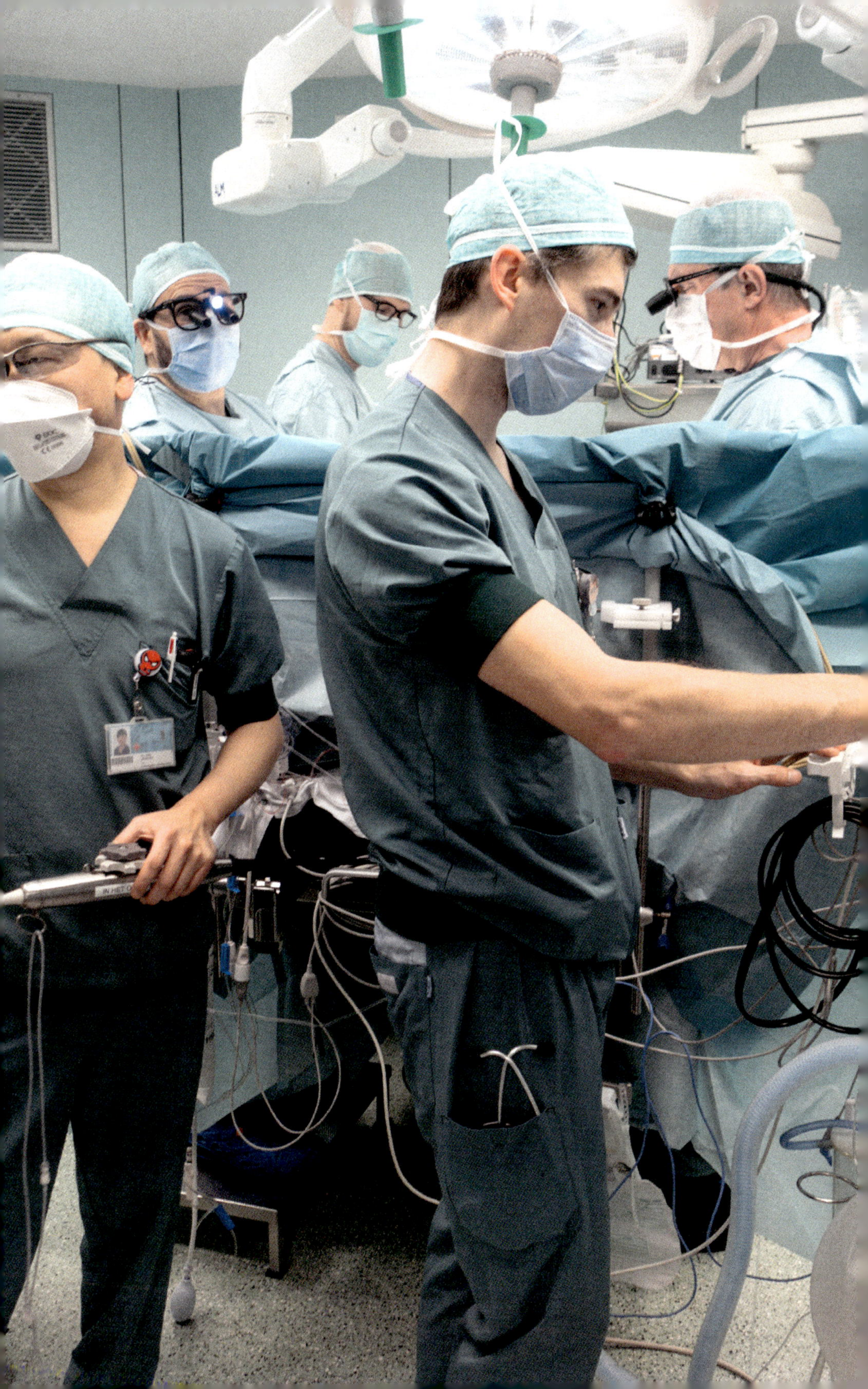

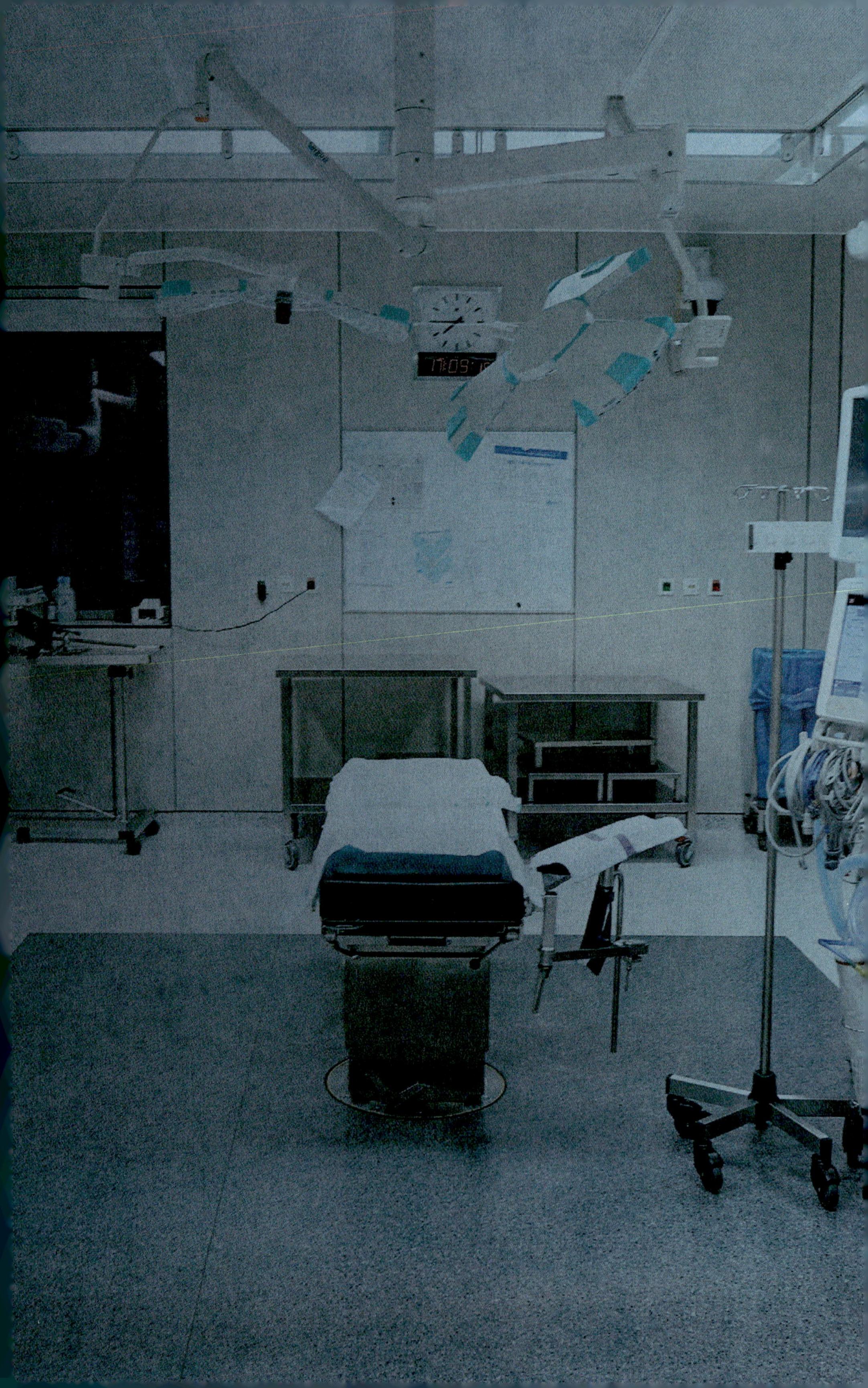

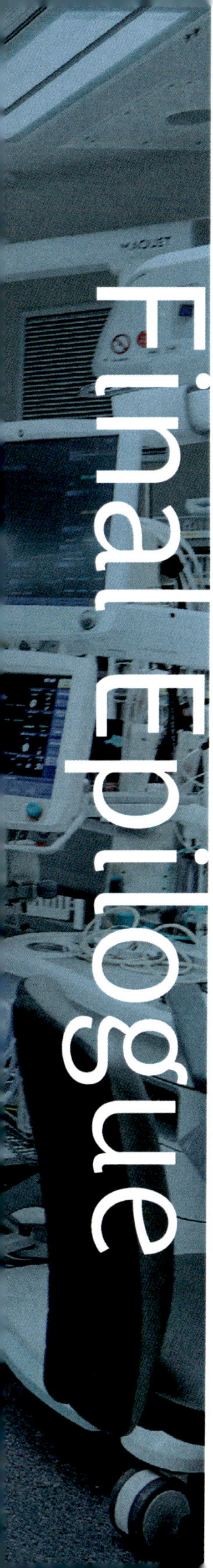

When the Room Is Quiet Again

At the end of the day, the operating room empties.

The instruments are gone. The anesthesia machine and its mechanical breathing system are silent again, standing where it stood that morning. Screens go dark. The floor is cleaned until it gives no hint of what happened there hours before.

If you walk in then, you would never know. You would not see the decisions that were made just a few minutes or hours ago. The moments when physiology struggled and was corrected. The tension that rose and settled again. You would not hear the alarms that alerted to the dangerous trends, or notice the interventions that prevented them from sounding.

Anesthesiology leaves very little behind. No incision to admire. No image to frame. No dramatic ending to retell. When we do our work well, the evidence is absence: the absence of catastrophe, the absence of pain, the absence of memory.

A patient wakes up. Breathing. Intact. Unaware of how close their body may have come to its limits. That is the positive outcome in the world of anesthesiology.

I have come to understand that this kind of work changes how you see the world. You learn to respect systems that hold under pressure. You learn that diligence matters more than brilliance, and that preparation matters more than confidence.

The responsibility does not end when the case does.

It follows you home. It shapes how you listen, how you decide, how you respond when things go wrong elsewhere in life. It teaches you that calm is not the absence of fear, but the ability to act despite it. That control is not dominance, but stewardship.

This book was never meant to explain anesthesiology in full. No book could. It was meant to make visible what is usually unseen, to slow time just enough to notice moments that pass without recognition. Over the years, I took mental notes, written notes, and photographs, capturing what unfolded quietly at the head of the bed. These pages are shaped by that accumulation of reflection, observation, and memory. They acknowledge a profession that does not announce itself, yet underpins everything modern medicine dares to attempt.

If you are not an anesthesiologist, I hope you leave with a deeper appreciation for the quiet trust you place in someone you may meet only once.

If you are a student, I hope you understand what this path asks of you, before you decide whether to take it.

And if you are an anesthesiologist, I hope this feels familiar. Not idealized. Not dramatized. Just honest. And for those who choose it, that is the privilege.

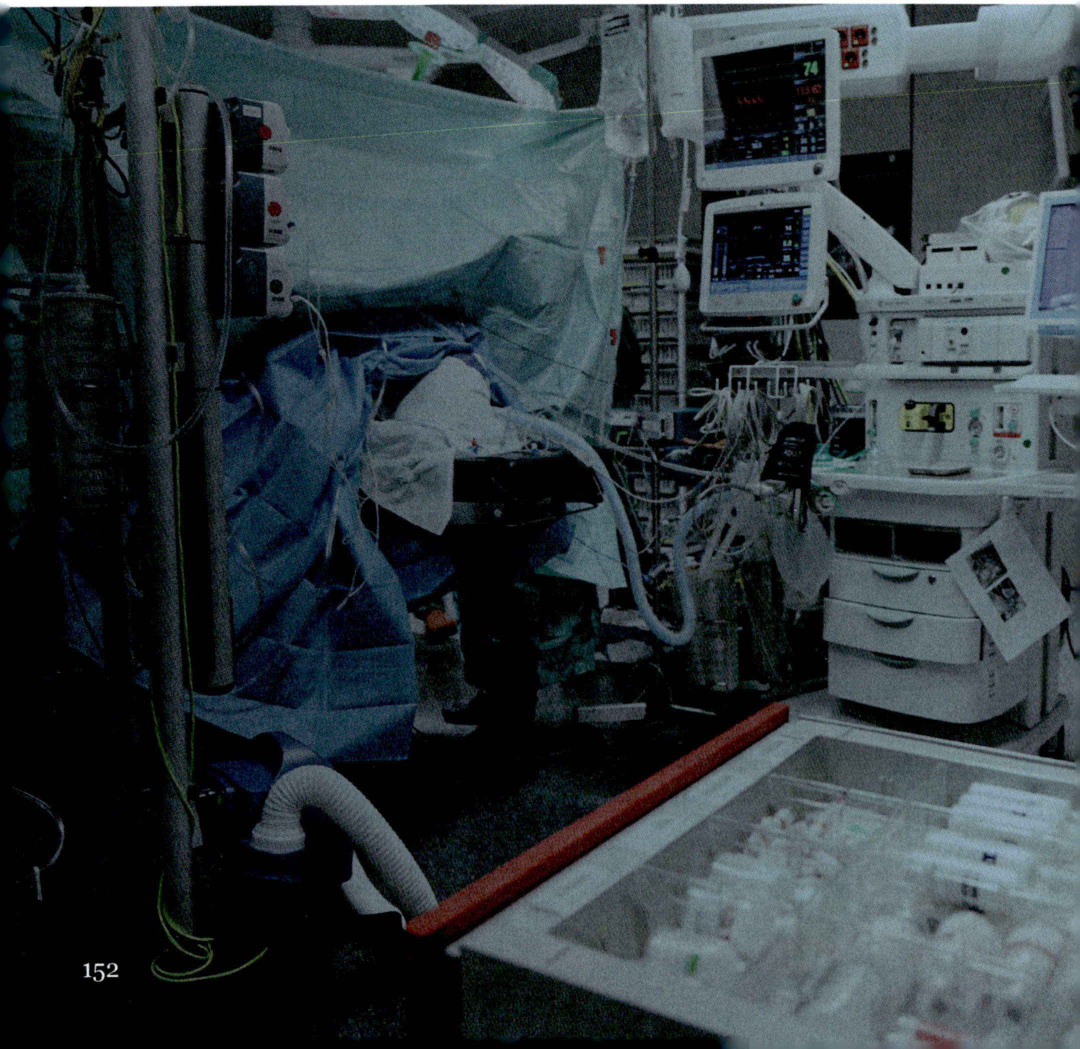

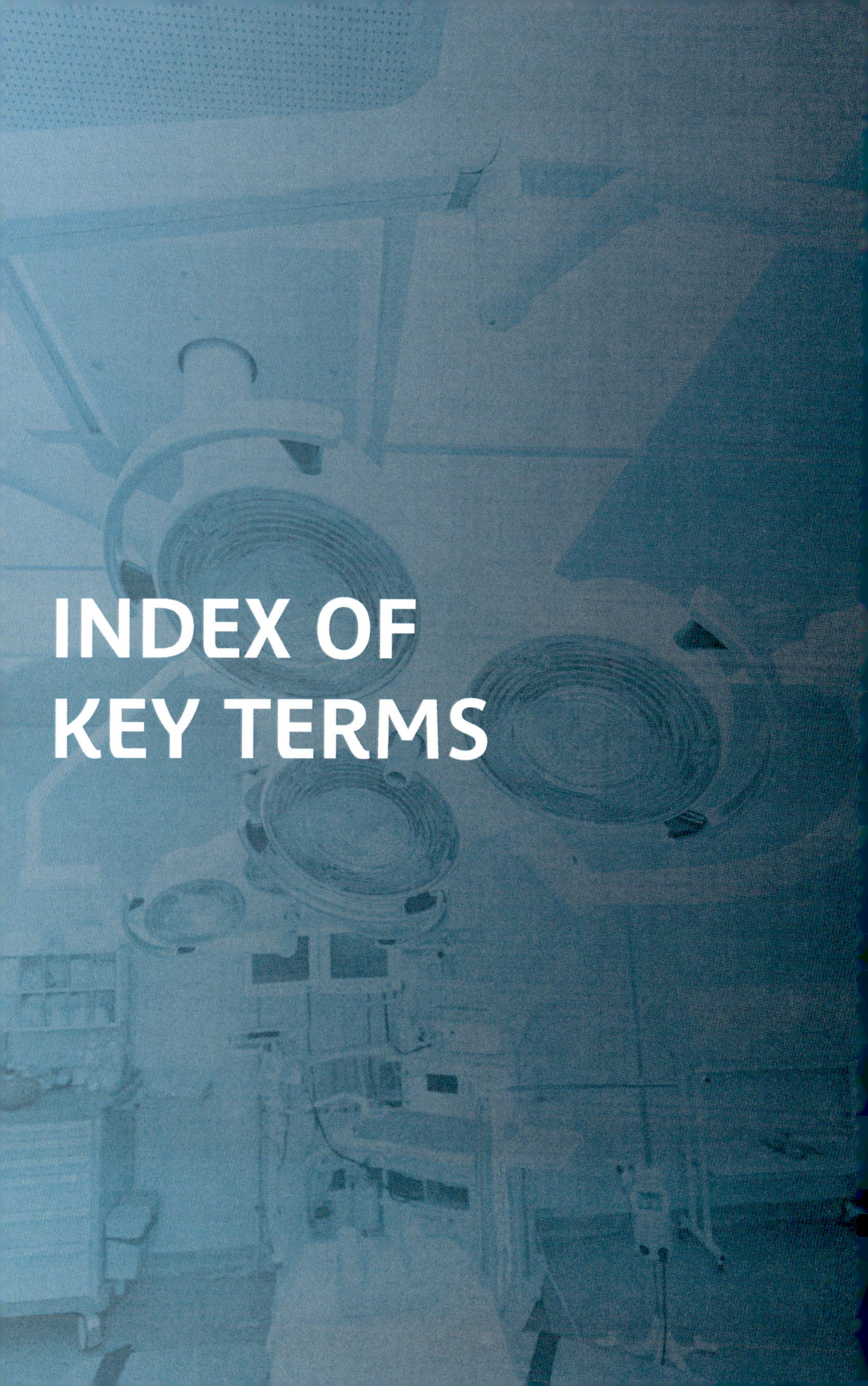

INDEX OF KEY TERMS